To Annie,

Your warmth and ... ... made spirituality is ...

You are magnifi... wonderfully blessed, and power fully endowed!

Great Things Happen Through You

Your Sisterfriend

Catrina

Peculiar Pain

*A Close Look at
Black on Black
Sexual Harassment
and Its Impact*

Patricia Wingard Carson

Motivational Institute, Inc.
P.O. Box 328712
Columbus, Ohio 43232

 KENDALL/HUNT PUBLISHING COMPANY
4050 Westmark Drive   Dubuque, Iowa 52002

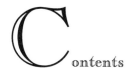

Contents

Foreword

Peculiar Pain is a story of a woman's fight for survival and respect in the workplace. Not since the nation witnessed the story of Anita Hill, and her experience at work with her supervisor Clarence Thomas has, a story been told that clearly and dramatically exposes sexual harassment in the workplace. The story of Patricia Wingard Carson is a detailed account of what many women across America are being forced to endure to keep their jobs and support their families.

Peculiar Pain is particularly poignant in its illumination of sexual harassment of Black women by Black men. The story captures the failure of one Black man's ability to handle his insecurities and his exercise of power over his female employee. The disrespect and humiliation meted out by this man is both sad and outrageous. But equally sad is the reality that this story is not unique nor rare.

It is only after sharing the author's story as it unfolds can one understand how this crime in the workplace creates thousands of victims each year in the nation. To do nothing enhances the crime and to underestimate its existence and impact encourages it.

Sexual harassment in the workplace between Blacks is no less despicable then among whites. But as a historically oppressed people it is ironically distasteful to see a Black man do this to a Black woman.

Peculiar Pain shows not only the devastating effects of sexual harassment in the workplace, but also gives guidance to victims as to how to best respond to this harassment. By giving the legal background of this issue and referral information for community services, the author provides others a foundation of understanding she lacked as a victim. Additionally, her final words to Black men expresses her pain and suffering but retains her love and faith in their greatness.

As a Black man I found that the strength and support of her husband, and other male family members, as articulated here, provides the understanding that this is not a story just negatively attacking Black men but rather one that painfully illuminates how too many of them are abusing their influence and power relative to Black women.

Patricia Wingard Carson shows us how to survive and how to fight back. Her spirit to make changes keeps her determined to stop the crime of sexual harassment in the workplace, and given where she has come from, such an effort is not impossible.

Jeffrey David Johnson
State Senator of Ohio - 21st District

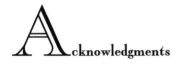

Acknowledgments

To my husband, "I love you and I sincerely appreciate you more than you'll ever know. Thank you, Jeff, for being a stabilizing force in my life and helping me to experience the strength of your manhood. With you I feel loved, balanced and safe.

Momma, (Ruby N. Jones) and Daddy, (Jeff Jones), the seeds of love and principles you planted in me have taken hold. Thank you for giving me *roots & wings.*

A special spiritual thank you to Tene', Marie, Adria, and Maisha, (Little Mai). Your intuitive support and input was always very timely. You never let me lose sight of the power of truth.

Reggie, your sincere brotherhood is what every sister needs in the workplace. Thanks!

An enormous thank you to all the prayer warriors whose prayers raised the standards against evil and brought down the strongholds: Momma Leon, Daddy Coy, Aunt LaVern, Aunt Ruth, Mom Earlene, Kimberly, Ella, Carla, Karen, and the entire Mt. Hermon Missionary Baptist Church membership, your prayers availeth much.

Judi and Mai, thank you for showing me that sisterhood is not always based upon color.

And to my sons, Dorian, Derrick, and Christopher, and my Godson, Ryan Coy Jones, may your spirituality keep you God centered and may you permit your inner light to guide your manhood and return you fully to internal Khamit... *a place and time when we were ruled by our Creator and acknowledged our devine heritage.*

To everyone and every organization who took time out to answer my sexual harassment questionnaire, thank you. Without your input, this book would be incomplete.

Delores, Corgie, Tene', Jeffery, and Monica, I love you. You are the best sisters and brother anyone can ask for.

Toni, Lynn, Sandra, Donna, Laura, Rhonda, Leslie, Deana, and all sisters who are afraid to speak out: Stand up and be heard!

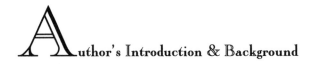

Author's Introduction & Background

The more I begin to share my experience of Black on Black sexual harassment with other Afrikan American women, the more my reluctance to write this book wore down. Many Black women I spoke with had scars of disappointment etched in their hearts and were unable to speak up because remembering was too painful. Some chose to put their experience of Black on Black sexual harassment behind them and hoped that it would never happen again. Many others never knew that it was alright to publicly speak out against this type of inter-cultural oppression.

I remember my first experience with being vocal against an issue I felt was important. I was in the 10th grade and a member of the Oberlin High School Marching Band. The name of our football team was the Oberlin Indians. Our mascot was a red-faced Indian with a hatchet and feather. The cheers we shouted were full of words like "scalp 'em", "massacre", "slaughter", and other violent verbs and adjectives. It never occurred to us that we were promoting negative images of Native Americans until my friend Monique, who was a Native American exchange student, spoke out against our mascot and cheers. Monique wanted our high school to choose another mascot or change the negative words in our cheers. She organized a sit-in. And I chose to participate in the sit-in along with a hundred or so other students. There was a lot of anxiety and mixed emotions surrounding this issue. Everyone who participated appeared to be anchored in their convictions, until the bell rang and the principal announced over the PA to clear the hallways at once. At first, no one moved. Then he warned us again. Only this time, he added that if the hallways were not cleared immediately, all classroom doors would be locked and the students who chose to remain in the hallways would be suspended. About twenty students got up and went to their classes, but not me. Monique was my friend and I had seen the hurt in her eyes and heard the conviction of her belief in her voice. I had to stay no matter what.

Then, like a clasp of thunder, there was a final warning bell and a loud authoritative voice demanding, "Leave immediately and return to your class or you will each be suspended!" More than half of the remaining students got up and left, but not me. There were about thirty of us who stayed and stood our ground. And as promised, we were marched into the office and one by one we were suspended. Our parents were called to pick us up.

Momma came and picked me up. On the way home she asked me what happened. She always allowed us to explain our behavior before she disciplined us. I told her about my friend Monique and how bad she felt about the things we said about her people in our cheers. I told Momma that I wanted to help Monique make a change. Momma listened very attentively and simply said, "It's important to stand up for what you believe, but you have to be prayerful about it. Sometimes it'll cost you more than you bargained. So make certain that what you believe in is good, just, and righteous. That way, God will always be on your side and fight your battle."

Momma's words stuck in my mind. Not only did she support my decision to help Monique, she helped me catch up with my missed school assignments while I was suspended. Everything worked out fine in that regard. Unfortunately, Monique did not succeed in changing the mascot or the cheers. But she made a lot of us think about the impact our actions can have on others. She gave me a deeper sense of compassion.

Now, almost 25 years later, I find myself still choosing to stand up for what I feel is good, just, and righteous. I've also learned that there will not always be a crowd to cheer me on. And that sometimes I'll have the support of family and friends and sometimes I will not. But still I must stand on the convictions my Creator places on my heart and be willing to face the challenges of my choice; For without challenge, there is no change.

In a small college town like Oberlin neighbors were truly neighbors. If my sisters or myself, brother, or cousins were caught doing things we weren't supposed to, we could count on being disciplined by almost any Mom or Dad in Oberlin. Talking back or being disrespectful to an adult was unheard of and was a punishable kid-crime.

Momma and Daddy kept us involved in numerous community and cultural activities. In the summertime Daddy worked a great deal as a construction worker. Momma chaperoned us everywhere. She built her life around her children and church. I don't know how she ever had time for herself.

There were six of us. My oldest sister, Delores, was married and lived in Chicago. Corgie, my second oldest sister, took tap dancing and flute lessons. Toni, my third oldest sister, took ballet and played the clarinet while my fourth and youngest sister, Monica, and I played the piano and took modern jazz dance lessons. Jeffrey, my only brother, was on the little league baseball team and took trumpet lessons.

Every Saturday after our daily baths, we got our hair washed and the girls had to line up to sit in what we called the "hot chair" to get our hair pressed with a hot comb and Royal Crown pressing oil. We had to be what Daddy called, "all gussied-up" for Sunday. Sunday was church day -- all day long. We were members of Christ Temple Apostolic Church and Elder Grady Benton was our pastor. He was very devoted to church and family and strong in the word.

Many times we went to Sunday school the next morning with a burnt ear or two. After Sunday school we went to morning service. After morning service we ate Sunday dinner that was prepared in the church basement or we ate at Grandma Leons. She and Grandaddy Coy were the only grandparents we had. They were the cornerstones in the family. After dinner, we went back to evening service. My favorite part was testimony service. I really liked listening to Sister Pearson testify. Sister Pearson was one of the mothers of the church. She would always give the most stirring testimonies. You could tell that she had been through a lot of trials and tribulations and learned to depend upon God a lot. Her testimonies could almost raise the hairs on your head, and it didn't matter to her that she didn't have a tooth in her mouth either. When she spoke and sang the praises of the Lord, everybody listened. She would open up her testimony with, "I love e-v-e-r-y-b-o-d-y!" Her words were always so spiritually charged and full of emotion. She would stretch and wave her arms up in the air shouting that she was on fire for Jesus! ...then with a happy, loud trembling voice, the rest of her testimony would began. "My soul's on fire... I thank God, I'm full of the precious Holy Ghost!" If it wasn't for the Lord, I don't know where I'd be. He has kept me when I couldn't keep myself. When I was sick and laying on my bed of affliction and the doctors had given up on me, He healed my body. But most of all, he saved my soul, and I thank Him, for e-v-e-r-y-t-h-i-n-g!"

Sister Pearson's favorite song was *'I'm on the battlefield for my Lord'*. Every Sunday she'd wear a little hat placed awkwardly on her silver-gray hair and sing the entire song as part of her testimony. And Every Sunday I got emotionally drawn into her words. Then for two Sundays in a row, I didn't see her in church. Later I found out that Sister Pearson had died. I remember thinking to myself how much I was going to miss her. I guess she lived what she sang about all those years. She praised God till the day she died. To this day, when I get still and quiet enough, I can hear Sister Pearson's high trembling voice singing,

> *'I'm on the battlefield for my Lord*
> *Yes I'm on the battlefield for my Lord.*
> *Well, I promised Him that I would serve Him till I die*
> *I'm on the battlefield for my Lord ....'*

Tuesday nights we went to young peoples meeting at church

and on Thursdays and some Fridays, my sisters, brother, and I, and three cousins, Cat, Betty, and Marsha, had choir practice. We were called the Wolfe singers. We were named after our Grandaddy Coy Wolfe. Momma and Aunt Ruth always stayed busy keeping our white cotton shirts bleached, ironed, and starched. Grandaddy Coy took us from one church revival to another throughout the state of Ohio and convinced every church we visited to listen to us sing. He would stand up during testimony and walk to the front of the church and start testifying on how good God was. He would be on a roll and everybody would be saying "Amen" and "Hallelujah". After Grandaddy saw he had them going, he would start talking about how good his youngins' could sing. He'd tell everybody that we were the Wolfe singers and that the Lord had blessed us to travel from church to church, singing His praises. He'd always say, "I'd like for you to listen to my grandchil'ren as they render an A and B selection. I love them so much I could just eat 'em up -- and sometimes I wished I had." The next thing we knew the whole church was clapping while we were on our way to the front of the church where we'd sing our hearts out for Grandaddy Coy -- many times without a piano. But the rthymn of hand claps and stumping feet, accented with the jingle of the tambourine was all we needed. The smile our songs brought to Grandaddy Coy's face was unforgettable.

It was good to grow up close and loved within an extended family community. However, in doing so, a false perception of the real world was created for my siblings and I. As time passed, one by one we became adults and left the comforts of home. Ignorant to what was in store, it wasn't long before life caught me on the blind side. In what seemed like a twilight of time, I went from a free-spirited child to a young mother with two sons, imprisoned by an abusive marriage and living in the suburbs of Chicago.

Daydreaming became my escape and cloak of protection. My sister Toni's spirit was so entwined with mine that we could feel each others internal pain or joy. We both attested to literally feeling our close spiritual connection. She says she feels me pulling on her for strength even though we are hundreds of miles apart. We wrote each other religiously, just like the sisters in the *Color Purple.*

It's funny, when we were kids, Toni and I were such opposites. She was the perfect example of what little girls are made of. Grace, charm, paper dolls, lace, ribbons, and pigtails. To her, femininity was a crown and she wore it well. As for me, I was totally unaware of what being a girl meant.

My favorite past-time was riding on the handle bars of my brother Jeffrey's, fat-wheeled bicycle. I paid no attention to Daddy's warnings about falling off and getting all scarred up. I wore my battle scars with pride and I rarely cried when I got them. I was a true baseball playing, tree-climbing, barefoot, tom-boy. Momma and Daddy felt pretty safe with allowing us to grow up in Oberlin. We were truly free to be children.

My sister, Corgie, nicknamed me, "Oogie", before I could even walk. Walking for me came pretty early. When I was about 9 months old, I traveled from by car from Oberlin to Alabama with my family. I'm told that the ride was long and hot. When we arrived in

Alabama and pulled up into Aunt Neil's drive-way, Momma lifted me out of the car and stood me by her leg. Momma said seems like I was so happy for my feet to finally touch the ground, that I took-off running and walking and haven't stopped since.

Eventually, I chose to escape my abusive marriage. With my youngest son Derrick, being weaned from the bottle, and my oldest son Dorian, being potty-trained, I ran away. I left behind everything I could not fit in two large plastic garbage bags. Once again, I decided to choose what I thought was good, just, and righteous. Little did I know that years of poverty were ahead of us. But with God and family, we survived.

Ten years after my divorce I obtained a college degree and my first real job with the Attorney General's office. Two years after that, I met an FBI Agent named Jeffrey Carson. It was unknown to me that we would continue to encounter one another and fall in love.

I was a part-time radio talk show host and Jeff was one of the guest I interviewed on my weekly show entitled, *Roadmap*. He was a man after my heart and went out of his way to prove his love to me. It worked! I found in Jeff, all the missing ingredients from the first marriage. The rest is history...

After about seven years in the workplace, I became an employee for the Court of Claims as a field coordinator with the Ohio Victims of Crime Compensation Program. My director and supervisor was a Black man. Little did I know that he was also to be my cross.

The story you are about to read, *Peculiar Pain*, is about my experience in the workplace with Black on Black sexual harassment.

It isn't a pretty story but it had a pretty tremendous impact on my life. Unfortunately, I've found it to be a familiar story for too many other Afrikan American women.

I tell this story in hope of helping to prevent others from experiencing the adverse effects this type of inter-cultural oppression can have. My greater hope is to help the victimizer or potential victimizer understand the impact of his or her actions.

My rough mountain climb experience taught me that it's not enough to just merely survive. You must prevail over circumstances that dare to rob you of your dreams.

In telling my story, I have made painstaking efforts to select words that convey its reality, with caution not to offend my readers. But please allow me to say this regarding the use of the word, "nigger", in this book. I do not condone or support the use of this word, nor is its use tolerated in my home or by my family.

It is used here at times in actual quotes from a man who evidently has internalized self-hatred and is perpetuating the worst of white-society's images of Afrikan Americans.

I use the word, "nigger", myself in my pain and anger as I felt betrayed, trapped and torn between my need for my job and my self-respect and fair treatment from a person who was not only my boss, but a man from my own culture.

Using this term to refer to my harasser, myself, and my co-worker is another indication of the destructiveness of the legacy of oppression in this country.

I hope I have succeeded in my efforts to get you to understand the brevity of damage sexual harassment creates.

Special discount rates are available when ordered in bulk quantities.
(614) 276-5155

For speaking engagements and or sessions on sexual harassment education and prevention, contact:
MOTIVATIONAL INSTITUTE, INC.
P.O. BOX 328712
COLUMBUS, OHIO 43232

AUGUST IS

SEXUAL HARASSMENT EDUCATION MONTH

For more information on implementation in your area and a free copy of the "Sexual Harassment Education Month Resolution", write to:
Patricia Wingard Carson, Founder
P.O. Box 328712, Columbus, Ohio 43232

PART I

THE STORY

Journal Entry   I

"Goddamit Patricia!" Bo yelled. "I's runs this her' Court! And if you don't get that through your thick skull," pointing his long, ashy finger in my face, "You'll find yourself out on the sidewalk looking for another job! You weren't nothin' before I brought you here! A nobody! Look at me! Do you understand that I signs ya paycheck? Me! I runs this her'! Not the Supreme Court Chief Justice, not the Supreme Court Judges, and certainly not fuck-up, Spuds! ME! Do you understand English?! Do you hear me? Speak up and answer me when I talk to you! I had big plans for you, but you just won't act right!" (All of this and I had no witness!)

(Thoughts)

> *God, I feel so numb. I can't even lift up my head -- it feels so heavy -- like lead. Oh, Lord, my tear ducts are walling up. I can't let him see me cry... and what does he mean by act right? Sex? That's what that bastard Arthur used to say after he beat me. Bo's a mean, sick, cruel, bastard, just like that first fool I was married to. How in God's name did I attract another fool like that into my life? When I finally ran away from Arthur to save my life, I thought God had healed and cleansed me from that abusive experience. And now, years later, here's the same demon looking me straight in my eyes again. Big Bad Bo! Lewd, carnal, and confused. Who in the world do you think wants you!? I wonder if he beats his wife? I wonder if she's scared to leave or take up for*

herself, like I was, when I was married to Arthur and enslaved to his abuse.

> *(What's wrong with me? Why am I just sitting here looking stupid and acting defenseless? Why won't I speak up for myself?)*

This nigga done lost his mind and I must have lost mine, sittin' here takin' this bullshit!

Journal Entry II

It's strange how Bo makes me feel like I'm a weak nobody. He's quick to remind me, "I runs this Court." Just last week he had high praises for my work and progress and made those comments to my co-workers and husband. Now I'm the brunt of his sexually explicit jokes. Every time he comes around me, I get ill. If the word n-i-g-g-e-r ever had any meaning -- he defines it. (Lord, I'm trying to stop using that word).

Bo always approaches me invading my personal space. His huge, round, egg-shaped body feels so overpowering. I can't stand it when he puts his hands on me. He's always touching me. His touch feels demonic, and his hands are like an octopus in heat always reaching and grabbing, touching me on my shoulders and manipulating me into his space, while his wanton eyes undress me -- he's totally thuggish. He dangles my job like a carrot on a stick in front of a rabbit. There's no doubt he wants to have me as his lover and the thought makes me nauseous. I feel like a trapped rabbit preyed upon by a hungry, vicious wolf. This is the highest paying job I have ever had and I enjoy it! After an abusive marriage, and more than ten years of poverty while struggling through college as a single parent, I felt like my sacrifices were beginning to pay off but this demonic bastard was trying to ruin it by taking it away. Because of what? --- sex! 'God help me ---give me strength to withstand this man, I prayed desperately.

Journal Entry   III

I'm the only female field coordinator for the Ohio Victims of Crime Compensation Program in the State. Part of my job is to advise innocent crime victims of reparations through this program, and here I am being victimized daily by the Program Director who was appointed by the Chief Justice of the Ohio Supreme Court. Not one employee in the entire Court of Claims seems to have the courage to stop this mad man. He constantly harasses women. But everybody acts as if they are too afraid to speak up. Maybe they too feel helpless. Maybe they hope that he'll get hit by a truck or something else befitting to the pain and anguish he causes others. It's embarrassing to be whipped in front of white folk by someone who looks like you. But consciousness, *not color*, makes a fool!

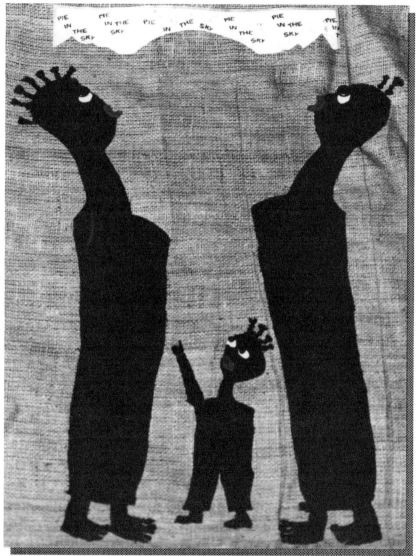

"Pie-in-the-sky -- in-the-sweet-by-and-by" I know the pie in the sky theory is a hoax... but it made it easier to bear the pain. So I kept looking up into the skies - - Looking to taste that pie theys keeps on a promisin' me.

Journal Entry IV

I try to ignore Bo and pretend that his abuse doesn't effect me, but he knows it does and I hate myself for allowing him to abuse me day after day after day. It's the same way I hated myself during my first marriage when I suffered the physical, emotional, and mental abuse from Arthur. I really thought I had overcome that part of me that permitted others to abuse and paralyze me with fear. I thought I had progressed beyond such stupidity. Why do I let people like Bo and Arthur cause me such pain over and over while I suffer in silence? This internal pain causes me much stress and I feel trapped. Every night, I cry and vow to speak up and make Bo stop hurting me. Each day I come home victimized, swearing that tomorrow will be the day I stand up for myself. But tomorrow doesn't come. My inability to take up for myself lets me know that I was just a broken vessel of sadness wrapped up in a facade of happiness. People look at me and think I've got it *goin' on*. If they could only see my shattered insides. Damn you Bo! Damn you to hell!

Journal Entry V

Somehow, Bo knows my hidden pain. Seems like a little devil sits on his left shoulder and whispers evil words into his ear that have the power to bind or break my spirit. His piercing eyes sit deep in their sockets waiting to penetrate my facade so he can control me. How? I don't know, but he does. Maybe I'm scared of him. Maybe I'm afraid he'll take my job away and I'll be poor again.

5

I fear that he might rape me or hit me if I say no to him when no one else is around. Every time he calls my name, my hands shake, and a knot wells up in my throat and blocks the natural flow of my breathing.

Journal Entry VI

Each day I get weaker and weaker. Too tired to keep trying. Uncontrollable tears seem to flow from my eyes for no apparent reason. I'm fighting depression but I feel like I'm losing. At night I

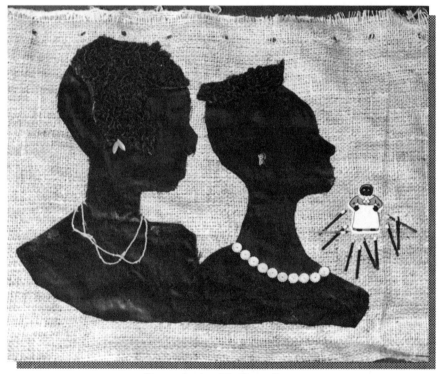

Remembering My Queenliness

toss and turn. My mind won't allow my body the rest it craves. I lay awake feeling alone and so angry, that a Black man would chose to sexually harass a happily married woman cut from the same culture cloth as he, but apparently not the same spiritual cloth. I feel betrayed and bewildered. I know I can't go on like this. I feel caught between a rock and a hard place. On one hand, I think of the struggles and rough mountain climbs it takes for Black men to become directors of companies and government agencies. I dare not betray my brother, *the Black man*, even if he abuses and harasses me... Bulls..t! That has to be bulls..t -- doesn't it? This man is slowly and methodically killing me! How can I not betray him if I'm to stay alive?

Seems like the hardest thing for me to remember these days is my queenliness. Everyday I have to burn the image of Aunt Jemina from my mind. I sometimes forget what I am, who I am, and whose I am. Daily I must confirm that through God, I am magnificently made; wonderfully blessed; and powerfully endowed!

I was taught that to speak out against my Black brother was taboo, so I struggle to maintain my cultural loyalty. On the other hand, a inner spiritual voice cries out, "Shun the very appearance of evil --", "Expose him! His consciousness of abuse has no color and his only allegiance is to his own flesh. This type of person is detrimental to the well-being of all mankind. This dilemma created a peculiar kind of pain within my spirit.

(Thought)

> *Biblical Paul was right when he wrote, in Ephesians 6:11-12, "Put on the whole armor of God, that ye may be able to stand against the wiles of the devil. For we wrestle not against flesh and blood, but against principalities, against powers, against rulers of the darkness, of this world, against spiritual wickedness in high places..." and so the struggle continues!*

Journal Entry VII

Writing helps me cope with my pain and empties my cup of grief when it overflows. Last night I tossed and wrestled for so long that I decided to get up and read and write in my journal. Afterwards, I prayed and meditated. I knew the next day I would again face the devil himself.

Journal Entry VIII

I'm a prayerful person, but now I find myself becoming more and more anguished in prayer. Today I had the nerve to interrogate God. "God, you know I have a burning need to know why I feel so helpless with Bo. Lord, why is my tongue, a tongue that is normally witty and fiery, not responsive to Bo's piercing, well-aimed, harassing words? Why does my tongue feel paralyzed? Why Lord, do you forsake me when you know I need you? Why Lord, do you allow this bastard to step on my pain and humiliate me in front of these white folk? Haven't I been through enough tests to prove my faith to you,

God? Is this my reward, humiliation from a Black man?

"Remember your promises to me God? Are you gonna keep your word or not? I'm not perfect, but I am a striver. Bo uses your name in vain practically everyday. He refers to his own mother, the womb that gave him birth, as a bitch, and you let him walk on me, your child! I don't get it! Are you asleep or what, God? Am I? Wake me up and deliver me from this nightmare! I don't know what to do, or say and I need my job.   My husband is being very supportive, but right now Lord, I don't even think he understands the hurt I feel inside. I feel withdrawn even from his touch. Making love seems to be the last thing on my mind. It is very difficult in the mornings to get up and get dressed to go work in Hell!"

"Now Lord, you said in your word that my enemies would become my foot stool and you've seen me through a past that was full of challenges, and you delivered me. You never left me through my years of poverty. You fed me and my kids and kept a roof over our heads, clothes on our backs and shoes on our feet. So I know you're able.

But this time, Lord, seems different. No matter how good of a job I do for this man, he curses me with his viperous tongue, touches me with his probing hands and pierces me with his evil eyes. I don't know how much more I can stand! Please, God! If you are there, and if you care anything about me, I need you NOW! I think I'm face to face with a demon!"

Journal Entry IX

Tomorrow I'm scheduled to attend a conference at Deer Creek. Bo directed me, Robert, and Lillian to attend so that we could help set up tables, disseminate literature and do other tasks incidental to conference planning. Bo told me, "After the Deer Creek conference, Patricia, you'll go with me to Cleveland to the National Association of Blacks in Criminal Justice Conference. Robert was scheduled to go but that's changed. We'll be staying overnight in a hotel in Cleveland." When he said overnight in a hotel, I got instant diarrhea, and almost lost total control of my bowels. I was petrified at the thought of being alone in a hotel with Bo!

The Deer Creek conference is scheduled to start pretty early. Bo had a room reserved for me at Deer Creek the night before the conference. I'm not too eager to be out at a resort all night with him lurking around. He has his way of using his authority to inch into my space. I wanted to avoid any opportunity of being alone with him, so I asked my husband, if he would take me to Deer Creek very early in the morning around 3:00 a.m. That way, I could arrive early, get dressed and be ready to perform conference assignments and hopefully, avoid Bo. Jeff agreed.

I packed and prayed, prayed and packed, but my thoughts kept looping over and over with a teasing, hollow message,... *I'm about to go into the den of iniquity with a crazy man... I'm about to go into the den of iniquity with a crazy man... I'm about to go into the*

10

den of iniquity with a crazy man........ Jeff saw my nervousness and grabbed and held me. He talked with me, comforted and encouraged me for hours. He's good at that sort of thing. When I first told him how Bo treats me, he was very angry and said he'd kick Bo's high-romped, rusty, black ass. I begged Jeff not to do or say anything. I wanted to be able to handle things and I stayed hopeful and actually believed that Bo would leave me alone. I was determined that he wasn't going to break me. Besides, Bo, the republican, is always bragging about how close he and former Cleveland Mayor, James Litchovich are. He said, "When Litchovich wins the upcoming gubernatorial election, he'll appoint me, the most progressive black republican in Ohio as one of his cabinet members." Since the election was right around the corner, I thought I could at least outlast Bo.

I was working and praying hard that Litchovich would win and Bo saw to it that I campaigned on behalf of Litchovich. I couldn't imagine anyone in their right mind appointing a demonic spirited man like Bo to be director over any agency. Bo appears to be dangerously unstable. He has no respect for God, and no allegiance to anything or anyone. He is bound by unjust laws and only seems to be interested in scratching the itch at the end of his penis. He seems to have sold his spiritual and cultural responsibilities for temporal, illusive carnal power. Chief Justice, Douglas J. Morton, certainly picked a good "field overseer", when he appointed Bo as Director of the Victims of Crime Compensation Program. Perhaps

11

the Chief Justice is also paralyzed by Bo. Whatever Bo's evil yoke-like spell is, only God and satan knows and only God's anointing power can break it!

As Jeff and I were driving to Deer Creek, my mind wandered back to one of Bo's cursing and yelling spells. I could see and hear his loud mouth as plain as day banging and pounding on his desk and pointing his long ashy finger at me after I had told him that I didn't appreciate him talking to me the way he did. It took me three sleepless nights to build up the courage to say that. In response, Bo told me, "This Court doesn't give a damn about your feelings!" Then he continued screaming, "Let me tell you something, Patricia, I runs this her'. I runs anything and everything I choose, including you! If I die right now and go to hell, I'll be running things down there. If I die and go to heaven, I'll run things there too!" He got himself so worked up, you could see the veins in his temple throbbing through the flesh wrapped around his bald, sweaty head, and the muscles around his upper lip twitching. At that moment, within my spirit, I realized that Bo acted like he was suffering from a mental problem or he was demon possessed. Without the light of God, he was destined to fall from his illusive mountain of success. It was just a matter of time. He actually thought he was omnipotent.

When we arrived at Deer Creek, Jeff walked me to the registration desk and made certain that everything checked out fine before he left me. We hugged and cuddled and he saw in my eyes my emotional dilemma. His assurance gives me confidence though.

Besides, I knew that all I had to do was say the word and Jeff would put Bo in check, man to man. But for reasons I can't explain, I held Jeff's rescue at bay. Jeff asked me if Bo ever put his hands on me. I hesitated too long in my answer. Right away he knew I wasn't telling him the whole story. I saw that *full-metal-jacket* stare in his eye, and pleaded with him to let me handle it and finally convinced him that I would be alright. I knew that if Jeff confronted Bo about harassing me, somebody would get hurt or Bo would treat me worse or fire me and we needed both our incomes to survive. Bo was a person to whom you never said *"no"*, nor did you suggest corrective behavior. His mental state did not allow him to handle those two responses very well. At any rate, I knew that God would never allow me a burden too heavy to bear. *But it sure did feel like God overestimated me this time.*

Jeff had to get back to work in Columbus. I dressed and prepared for the conference. I hadn't slept the night before the conference and I was beginning to feel a little tired. I began to sing a tune remembered from my childhood church days to give me some energy. The words meant so much to me. Momma use to sing this song at the kitchen sink all the time. I wonder if she felt troubled all those times? I wondered if she ever got tired and worn. She always acted so strong! Perhaps she was looking for strength in the words she sang and my young mind could not comprehend her cry. They protected us so much, she and daddy, from the cruelness of the world. Perhaps too much... I could hear her singin' in my mind, I could feel her believin' in my heart...

> *What a friend we have in Jesus, all our sins and grief to*
> *share.*
>
> *What a privilege to carry, everything to God in Prayer.*
>
> *Oh what peace we often forfeit, oh what needless pain*
> *we bear.*
>
> *All because we do not carry, everything to God in*
> *prayer....*

She'd sing it over and over again, then shout praises of thanksgiving while she finished cleaning. It was common for us to see Momma on her knees early in the morning, praying the prayers of salvation and protection for her children. No doubt God knew her well for she talked to God all the time, out loud, wherever and whenever she thought on God's goodness. The thought of God's goodness would get into her bones and send an electrical shock throughout her body and she would fling her hands straight toward the heavens and break out into another gospel as tears streamed down her face, singing with the deep conviction of her faith...

> *When I think of the goodness of Jesus and all He has done*
> *for me, my soul cries out hallelujah, praise God for saving*
> *me!*

..then she would call all her children's names one by one and tell God about us, thank God for us, and make God promise to keep us safe from any hurt, harm or danger. I remember Momma's tears of

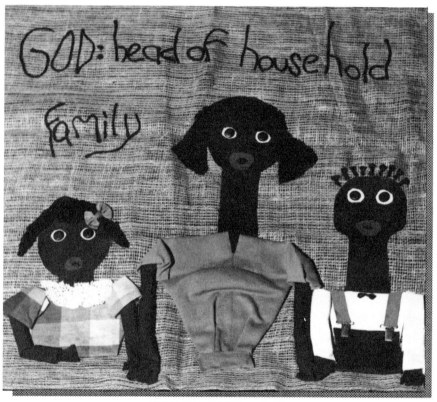

GOD: Head Of Household

concern that God would never leave or forsake her children. She loved every bone in our bodies and every hair on our heads, and she told God so. Momma was so fervent that God could not help but hear her plea.

I *know* Momma's prayers are sincere and are answered. Even as adults, my brother and sisters, and I feel Momma's prayers all around us, protecting and preparing. I get strength and assurance when I think of Momma's faith. She's truly a prayer warrior and I can't wait to tell her about Bo, so that she can tell God!

Although I hummed the songs of my mother that made my spirit uplifted, my physical body was in pain. My lower stomach was cramping and I felt like my period was going to start. It wasn't time for my period for another two weeks. I was upset and my stomach was probably reacting to the stress.

As I looked in the mirror to put on my mascara and I caught a glimpse of my own eyes, I captured a peek at the little, frightened, child inside of me. There I was, all alone and face to face with Patricia, without the facade. I began to stare at my inner self. As I stared, I felt an uncontrollable fear force its grip on my solar plexus. Warm tears began to fill my eyes until they burned and overflowed down my cheeks slowly filling the corners of my mouth. I could taste the saltiness of my pain. I didn't fully understand why I was crying so hard, but I do remember feeling so very helpless, alone, and afraid. I think I cried because I saw a grown woman who had given her peace and joy over to the hands of a handkerchief-head, *nigga man.* I saw a woman who had broken the barriers of poverty, struggled to graduate from college while raising two sons for ten, long, sacrificial years. For ten years I had kissed all kinds of ass to survive. For ten years I wore thrift-shop clothes and hand-medowns. For ten years, I walked, caught the bus or bummed rides. For ten years, I jumbled my bills, sometimes, sitting in the dark and not having a stove to cook on, or having my electric on and eating oatmeal 3 times a day in exchange for keeping on my gas so that me, Dorian, and Derrick could take warm baths in the winter time. Many cold winter nights, we slept in a twin sized bed piled with every blanket in the house, all scrunched up together so that our body heat could keep us warm. And when the cold bite of the morning came, we scurried around like little chipmunks getting dressed. I'll never forget the time we almost got evicted because I didn't have $10 to pay my rent in full... a measly ten dollar bill. That struggle of poverty made me and my sons pretty close and very protective of one another. I couldn't let them know how Bo was hurting me. It wasn't their battle and they would want to confront him. My youngest son, Christopher was still in school and I didn't want my problems to interfere with his school grades. I didn't want Bo's evil persona in their atmosphere at all! So as best as I could, I kept silent about my pain around them.

Ten long years of hell and humiliation just to arrive at the finish line and run into a mental bastard. What was suppose to be a small measure of success ended up as a sad malady, a Black woman unjustly mistreated by a Black man. I take that word back, Bo's not a Black Man, he's by all definitions, *a nigger!* "'Nigger', is an attitude, not a color," my Aunt Vern use to say. She'd tell anybody that a "nigger" ain't always black!

I found myself talking out loud to God, *"Lord, help me help you, to help me."* As I dropped to my knees, the strangest words formed on my lips, "God, please heal Bo. Soften his hard old, wicked heart." As the last word rolled off my lips, I was captured in what felt like a frozen moment of truth. Truth etched upon my heart a vicarious experience. In that moment, I felt Bo's pain above my own. All of a sudden, I knew how terribly Bo disliked himself. How lonely he felt inside because nobody genuinely liked him. It was as if our spirits exchanged places to create compassionate understanding in my heart. To a racist, white individual, Bo was a *"good nigger"* who hated other Black people and who was more than willing to carry out hideous tasks against his own people for a slab of bacon. To Blacks, he was an obnoxious overseer with a whip too eager to please his master! To women, he was a nightmare...! In his search for love, he was totally lost. He used hate to try to find love. I asked God to give me the strength to endure my lesson and the wisdom on how to embrace it.

> *"Lord let my light shine and make my enemy my footstool.*
> *Through my faith, I must prevail. Lord, Thy will be done.*
> *Yes, Lord, My Soul says Yes Lord."*

With that prayer, I finished getting dressed and left to do my assignments just as Master Bo ordered.

As I sat at the registration table next to Lillian, the public information officer of the Court, I stared at her lily white skin and her light brown hair that she always kept neatly styled in a page boy. I inwardly wished I was comfortable enough to confide in her. I remember when I was in the 5th grade how I wanted to be Debbie Helkins. She was white and seemed to have everything I wanted - long bouncy pig tails, the teacher's love and acceptance; even the story books we read in school had pictures of little girls and boys that looked like her. She had pretty clothes and lots of friends and freedom. Guess I was going through an identify crisis. There was not much in school for me to identify with. Thanks to the confidence Momma, Daddy, and the rest of my family put in me, I got over that self-hate crises. But even now I felt myself craving for what Lillian appeared to have -- the freedom to be. I wanted to tell her that Bo was sexually harassing me. I wanted her to feel my pain and have compassion. I wanted her to see how much I was hurting. But she could not see the real me for my color. Besides, her sarcastic attitude made her seem unapproachable and far from being sensitive to my well-being.

Before I rejected Bo's sexual advances, he told me how impressed he was with my skills, and that he was grooming me to replace Lillian as the public information officer for the Court. Bo said that Lillian did not have very good people skills and her lack of public relations skills was bad for the Court. I felt that I had walked into the middle of an old battle. I also think Lillian's ears got hold of Bo's words and intent. She frequently withheld pertinent information from me. On one occasion, Bo told Lillian to train me on a computer program she had been instrumental in designing. She did not like that at all.

I told Bo about Lillian omitting important steps and information in showing me how to operate the computer program. All he had to say was, "I don't care how your ass gets the information, just get it!" Conflict and confusion seemed to fuel his soul. I wouldn't have been surprised if he had told Lillian one thing and me another just to sit back and watch the fireworks. When I asked Lillian about keeping information from me, she responded with a sweet, sarcastic apology.

Bo had taken a couple of other projects previously assigned to Lillian prior to my coming on board and gave them to me to finish. She pretended it didn't bother her, but I could tell it did. She was vindictive and her sharp comments were too frequent and full of viper's venom. Still, I put forth my best efforts to courteously accommodate her "smart-mouthed" responses, to no avail.

On the other hand, Lillian appeared to be a very disciplined but agitated person. She told me that she was once extremely overweight, and through exercise, and diet, she was able to lose a lot of weight. I admired her discipline, but didn't appreciate her attitude. Not once did I argue or fail to cooperate with her. I figured if she knew better, she'd do better. Maybe she never had a personal, pleasant, or intelligent experience with an Afrikan American. Maybe she believed the negative images that society painted and placed all Blacks. I was determined to be a positive Black experience for her. On the other hand, maybe she was a shepherd for wolf Bo, luring an innocent lamb (me) to slaughter.

Anyhow, after Lillian conveniently kept forgetting to tell me about important steps in operating the computer program, I asked her to write the instructions down step by step. Straight and to the point, I said, "Lillian, when you show me the steps to operate this program, you always seem to leave out important steps and when I follow your instructions, it never works out correctly and Bo is under the impression that I am not following your directions, when you and I both know that I am. He's expecting me to be proficient at this, soon. Are you doing this on purpose?" Her sweet, yet bitter response, "Oh Good heavens, no. I just really forgot to mention it." *Right, I thought!*

Still, I found myself wishing I had the peace of mind she appeared to have. I often wondered if Bo harassed her the way he harassed me, or if I took her place? Her superior attitude made her too unapproachable to ask or confide in. Besides, she seemed to enjoy watching a Black man mistreat his Black sister.

Journal Entry X

Lindsey, Bo's secretary, is an interesting person. People in the office said that she was fair game for any man in the office. To me, it didn't appear to be that way. She did smile and sometimes laugh at Bo's sexually explicit jokes and comments he made about her though. Lindsey did not seem bothered by Bo's behavior. I know people react differently when a person makes insensitive comments about them. It reminds me of the words from a song, *"Tears Of A Clown, When There's No One Around".* Sometimes, wearing a facade helps you survive and helps you keep your job.

Bo used Lindsey several times as the brunt of a sexual joke or comment. Once he said, "Lindsey, you sure look good with that donut hanging out your mouth." (The donut was oblong-shaped). He said it with a sexual undertone to imply his infatuation with oral sex. It sounded very degrading. On another occasion, in our morning staff meeting, Bo told a sexual Saint Peter's Day joke and Lindsey was the brunt. She just laughed. It's difficult for me to understand why another woman would outwardly perpetuate sexual harassment. Maybe there was more to what I saw and heard. Maybe Lindsey was just trying to keep her job like me. It was hard to tell. She was too close to Bo for me to risk betrayal had I confided my pain. She and Lillian both had been there longer than me and in my emotional distress, I could not find the strength to take the chance at being betrayed by them. So I remained silent and did not share my pain with either of them -- I couldn't.

Journal Entry XI

Robert, the other field coordinator for the Victims of Crime Compensation Program, was a well-mannered sensitive Black man. He knew about Bo's desire to "get with me". Robert was there for me when I would break down and cry after Bo's brow beatings and sexual innuendoes. Robert knew how to make me laugh when I felt pain and humiliation. He stayed focused on doing whatever Bo asked him to do. Bo didn't talk to people like they were human beings. His ways were very ugly!

"Sister, Sister", is what Robert nick-named me. I guess because he looked after me like a sister and tried to protect me from Bo's cruelness. We worked very close together. We were both Bo's victims. Bo thought that Robert was his flunky and I was his sexual object. So much for friendship and professionalism based on race. *Yeah, right!*

Robert and I joked around sometimes to lessen the pain and referred to ourselves as 'field niggers' instead of field coordinators for the Ohio Victims of Crime Compensation Program. That's certainly what Bo tried to make us feel like.

Robert's a family oriented, tall Afrikan American man from East Cleveland. He grew up with my husband's cousins in East Cleveland. Robert and I are anchored in God, family, culture, and community. Bo envied us for that. If Bo saw Robert and I getting along too good, he would call us into his office and give us the "Bo Gilyard Speech", on how to conduct ourselves.

I told Robert that I felt sorry for Bo because he seemed so unhappy with himself and angry with life in general. Robert told me Bo's happy, he's just mean. "Being mean makes Bo happy. The meaner he is the happier he is. If you start feeling sorry for him, he'll just misuse you even more," Robert said. At first, I couldn't understand Robert's words, but as time passed, it became quit apparent, that meanness to Bo was a climatic experience.

Journal Entry XII

Bo had a "drum major's instinct". He had a strong desire and need to feel important, to be first, and to be in charge. And he did this at the expense of humiliating other people he deemed as insignificant. Bo often boasted that one day he would be governor of Ohio. He told us that he would be in charge of this state's affairs, then he would run things his way! I had to listen to his plans, dreams, abuse, sexual jokes, name calling, ego tripping and theories on how and why being a black Republican really pays off. He said, "Most Blacks are what I call dumb nigger Democrats. They don't have the political savvy I have." Some of the comments that would burp from his vulgar mouth during staff meetings were so embarrassing to anyone with allegiance to culture, common sense and intelligence. His false sense of superiority was fueled by his thwarted perceptions of others. To him, nobody was right, good, or worthy of praise, but him. If they were, it was because they kissed his ass or psyched him into thinking they admired him. He made more ethnic and racial slurs than a Klansman. He made more sexual slurs than a caveman. He indicated that the Republican party accepted Blacks like him because he possessed a superior mind. He had no college degree, no good human relations skills, no positive managerial skills and no positive comments for other Blacks.

Once I approached Bo concerning the racial breakdown of

reparations (monies) awarded to innocent victims of crime. I was told around 87% of the $74,000,000.00 awarded had been awarded to white victims of crime and only about 13% had been awarded to black and other non-white innocent victims of crime. The reparations awarded were at a serious disproportion.

I very cautiously suggested to Bo that our agency was not adequately informing individuals in the inner-city of these available funds. I drafted a plan to create a multi-cultural awareness campaign targeting the inner-city community. I have been a T.V. and radio talk show host, newspaper columnist and magazine columnist and I have strong community ties and involvement. Therefore, I had the resources to help make this project very successful. I was very excited about the possibilities. I advised Bo of community events and shared unfortunate circumstances that happened in the inner-city community where our agency could be helpful to innocent victims. After sharing this plan, Bo was silent for a moment. Then with a deviant and devilish stare from his beady eyes, he said, "I decide the direction for this program! Me! Now get back to work! You're not getting paid to think," he growled. "You need to concern yourself with keeping your husband happy." I was so embarrassed and humiliated, without emotion, I said, "Yes, sir." and went back to work. Once again, I left King Bo's office feeling like an insignificant ant that had just been smashed on a city sidewalk. The pain was so swift and sharp, I didn't have time to say, *"Ouch!"*

Journal Entry XIII

One week later in a meeting, Bo mentioned (as if he came up with the idea) that he wanted me to contact inner-city community agencies and think of creative ways to promote our program at upcoming inner-city events. He cited the same resources and plan almost exactly as I had earlier advised him. He acted as if it was a fresh and new thought that had emerged from his round, bald head. I accommodated his ego and said, "Yes, sir, I'll get on it right away." My primary concern was helping victims and promoting the program. Who cares who came up with the idea. So, I smiled and thought to myself, "This is going to be an impressive and successful program. I'll prove to him that I can do a great job. If he would stop harassing me, it would be less stressful."

I immediately got the agency involved with the United Negro College Walk-a-thon. The logistics officer of this event is a good friend of mine so I contacted Charles to work out the details of our agency's involvement. (Bo assigned me to work on the project alone).

On the Saturday morning of the UNCF Walk-a-thon, I was up at 5:30 am to ready myself for the march. As the marchers left the starting point, I passed out over 1,000 Ohio Victims of Crime Whistles and Brochures. The walkers blew their whistles zealously during their walk, and I was able to engage in numerous conversations with UNCF participants and tell them about the program. People gave me information about upcoming community events. As expected, the Walk-a-thon was successful and was a good start for our agency's positive involvement.

Later in the week, I was able to give out brochures and whistles at Greenbrook Community Outreach Center. I conducted volunteer motivational training and self esteem counseling at this outreach center. Greenbrook is considered to be one of the highest crime rate areas in Franklin County. I also asked a friend who served as program director for a local urban radio station, if Bo could be a guest speaker on her hour long, live call-in radio talk show to inform the inner-city of the available funds, and how to apply for reparations. She said yes.

Bo appeared on the hour-long, call-in radio show. After which, he was presented with the *Citizen of the Week Award* from WCKX Radio Station. From that presentation, Bo received a proclamation of acknowledgment from the State House of Representatives.

Needless to say, the Ohio Victims of Crime Compensation Program was on a roll in the Black community. I was permitted to have the creative input necessary to help make it happen, only because nobody knows Bo and he needs me to bridge the gap for him in the Black Community. He probably would have me shot after I've outlived my usefulness to him, just like in the movies.

As an Executive Committee Member of the N.A.C.C.P. , I have direct involvement with several community agencies. One day, while reading our local paper, I learned that an innocent little 10-

year-old Black male child was killed in a drive-by shooting while sitting on the steps of his mother and father's neighborhood carry-out. He was shot in the head. His parents were forced to close the store to make arrangements and attend their child's funeral services. [Imagine the sorrow associated with the sudden death of one's child]. I immediately wrote down ways the program could help this family. I asked Bo if he would consider being involved in informing the parents about monies available from the Ohio Victims of Crime Compensation Program to aid their financial loss. Once again, he ignored the idea and told me to get back to work. This time I felt a need to spiritually and ceremonially kiss Bo's butt, and suck up to his ego. I tried very hard to persuade him that it would be the right thing to do and that there would be a lot of publicity and media coverage. [It's a shame that inner-city people, especially Black people knew little or nothing about the Ohio Victims of Crime Compensation Program, and I felt it was my duty to tell them].

I kept using the word "publicity" in my efforts to convince Bo that we should contact the family. As I kept saying "publicity", I could see his eyes come to life. He still told me to get out of his office and get back to work. I smiled as I thought of him drooling at my kept mentioning "publicity". I knew the word publicity pricked his pointy, little ears as he envisioned his name in media "headlines". In the meantime, I telephoned a friend who was involved in putting together a community march against crime which focused on the 10-year-old's death. I mentioned Bo's name to him and he said, "Bo who? I never heard of him. Who did you say this guy was?" I explained the program again and told him more about Bo's position. Finally, he said he would promote the program, not Bo.

The media follow-up about the murder of the 10-year-old child was still making big news headline. Bo had a sudden change of mind about getting involved with this project. He called me into his office and asked me if I could still arrange to get him involved with the community march against crime. I said, "Yes," trying to hide my excitement. I contacted the necessary people got all the details for Bo.

On the following Saturday, Bo and I arrived at the march in different cars and parked. We assembled and met with the rest of the marchers. Community leaders attended the march in full force. There were councilmen, councilwomen, state representatives, senators, ministers, N.A.A.C.P. officers, community activists and many concerned citizens. Various forms of media came out to cover the event.   WCKX Radio, who has a good track record of involvement with community events, set up a live radio broadcast. The march route went directly through the crime and so called gang-infested neighborhood where the 10-year-old was gunned down. The march ended at the store steps where the murdered child sat when the unidentified gunmen drove by in a car and fired the fatal shot into this innocent young man child.

"Such tragedy, sorrow, and Godlessness."

Prior to this community march, Bo seemed nervous about

29

being involved. He said he didn't know too many people in Columbus' Black Community. I tried to assure him that everything would be fine. His real concern was being around all those "ignorant niggers", as he often put it. I really couldn't understand why this man hated and mistrusted everyone who was of the same hue as he.

When we approached the crowd, I was greeted and embraced by many politicians and community leaders. Not one person, I mean absolutely nobody knew Bo. It was apparent that Bo was "a stranger in the hood". I introduced him and the program to many participants. To me, everything seemed to be going smoothly, but I could feel Bo gradually becoming pissed-off because he was not the center of attraction. Nobody realized his need for importance but me. Only I knew he was an ignored, ticking, time bomb waiting to explode.

As everybody listened and got instructions for the March, I could hear Bo grunting under his breath as if his thoughts were trying to break into words. People from all walks of life participated. There was even a trumpet player blowing away as if he were bringing down the walls of Jericho. The march began and ended as scheduled at the store front.

At the store front, participants stood at attention while listening to various speakers address the issues of crime, gangs, and violence in the inner-city. I took pictures, and circulated whistles and brochures as earlier instructed by Bo. Although Bo was not scheduled to speak, but I knew the WCKX's Program Director and the DJ that was operating the radio live remote, so I quietly took the liberty of asking Bo if he would like to say a few words over the air to thousands of listeners. He smiled, lit up, and growled with a graveled whisper, "Yeah." I told him I'd see what I could do to make it happen.

I approached Frank and Rick and told them about Bo and the program. Then I asked them if my boss could have some air time to tell their listening audience about the program. Rick reminded me that Bo was not scheduled to speak, but said, "Patricia, since I know you, I'll let the brother have a few minutes of radio air time to talk about the program. "Thanks Rick, I owe you one," I said.

Bo had a "lost but eager" look on his face as I walked back over to him. He was happy when I told him that he would be allowed to speak. I dared not tell him that nobody knew who the hell he was. I could literally see his ego growing before my eyes, as he said, "See, I'm more popular than you'd like to think, Patricia." His entire countenance and appearance changed. He was all smiles as he grabbed the front of his pants and yanked them up over his round belly several times to accommodate his high-romped frame. [Why he likes having his pants wedged in his crack is a puzzle to me]. I was so glad that Frank and Rick said yes, because I would have had hell to pay if the answer had been no.

Bo spoke to the crowd and radio audience as if he was speaking from the steps of Capitol Hill. Boy, this 'negro' loved to think he was important. He says that he's a better speaker than Jessie Jackson-- *Right!* I continued to take pictures and pass out brochures.

After Bo finished speaking, and received his applause, he walked over to me and leaned very close to my face. I freaked. I thought the fool was getting ready to kiss me, but instead, he whispered in my ear, "Put the camera away and stop taking pictures of these dumb, ugly, niggers. Let's Go! Now!" Although I was use to his lack of appreciation and unpredictable behavior, and even though no one else heard him, I felt embarrassed for him being part of my culture. He had his spot in the lime light and now his compassion quickly dwindled back to its reality - nothingness, selfishness, and evilness. He's a strange beast.

I left with him as he demanded before he became a bigger embarrassment. As we walked, Bo said that we had to go out to lunch and have a debriefing of what we achieved today. When was I going to get rid of him? A debriefing could have and should have waited until Monday when we got back to work. He was in no mood to entertain that suggestion. He insisted that I ride with him. I had no more sense than to go along with him.

We went to a restaurant located right around the corner. Upon arrival, the waitress ushered us past two Black men. I knew both of them very well. One was an attorney, Harry Thomas and the other was his business partner, Joseph Valentine. They were both good, responsible Black men. I remember having mixed feelings as

I approached them. Everything appeared to move in slow motion. When I looked at them, I probably had a strange expression on my face. I was happy to see them because it had been a long time since our paths had crossed. At the same time I knew if they demonstrated happiness when greeting me, I would be subjected to Bo's ill reaction, then I would have to listen to his rendition of his greatness.

As we slowly approached their table, I strained my thoughts so hard that I felt my temple jump. I was trying to telepathically tell them not to make a fuss over me. It didn't work! As Joseph always did, he stood and greeted me with a warm smile and Christian-like hug. Harry did the same. Unbeknownst to them, they had just triggered the psyche of a mad man. I was too stressed for words. But for once, I put my fears of what may happen aside and said to myself, "What the hell. Forget Bo! He's not going to control this warm moment in my life today; These are my friends and I'm going to be happy to see them because I am!" With that self-empowering thought, I reciprocated their greetings with the same warmth that they were given. I introduced them to Bo and tried to elevate his existence in their minds by boasting a bit about the importance of his position and the program. They shook his hand and presented themselves as the gentlemen I knew them to be. Then, Bo and I took our seats. We ordered our food. I ordered something very light so that I could finish quickly and get the hell out of Dodge. Bo ordered a heavier meal. When he did that I knew I was in for at least an hour of his grief. Before he took one bite, he began ranting and raving about "niggers". He said, "Niggers in Columbus are zeros. How do you put up with such nonsense, Patricia?" He glared back over to Harry and Joseph's table, and mumbled, "Like those two niggers over there. They think they're big shit. I don't think they care too much for me." I sarcastically responded, "Perhaps they don't know how important you are boss." To which he gleamed and said, "Yeah, they don't know me, yet." He was so blind with his own false superiority that he didn't hear the truth of my sarcasm.

(Thoughts)

Thank God they don't know you! Because if they had the smallest idea of how you're disrespecting me, they would probably kick your ass. There are more Black men in this world who know how to respect themselves and their sisters than there are lost souls like you. What baffles me is how Black men like you get into positions of authority. Have you always been this way or did your lose your sense of balance on your climb up? Besides, Bo, you're only a legend within your own mind. At the pace you're going, nobody would even weep at your funeral. Some would spit on your grave. You wish you were half the man either one of them are. Please, fool, eat your food so that I can get the hell out of your face and back to my family. You ain't nothin' but a speck -- a fly in a bucket of buttermilk, as my daddy use to say. And as long as your mind keeps playing tricks on you about your superiority over other people, you'll remain a speck. Your words are empty and your good deeds are non-existent. You should worry more about your soul and salvation, not material gain. It's blinding you and robbing you.

The next few days, there was more news coverage on the march against crime and violence. The media continued to mention the innocent killing of the 10-year-old child. Bo must have been keeping up with the news coverage because he called me into his office and asked, "Patricia, do you think I could *milk this thing* for more publicity?" I asked him what he meant. He asked, "What if I make a media announcement that my agency is going to help the bereaved parents cover their out-of-pocket expenses, which would include funeral cost and shit like that? Do you think we can get some mileage out of that?"

I knew his heart was not in the right place but I also knew that these people could really use the financial help, so I silently asked God to deal with Bo in a way that he would know to fear the raft of the universe. Then I said, "I think giving those parents financial assistance would be an excellent way to promote your program within the Black community.

Arrangements were made for the bereaved parents of the 10-year-old to come in and apply for reparations. Bo made certain that the affair turned into a big media blitz. The news stations were contacted and they wanted to cover the event. When they arrived, Bo told me to stay in the back in my office, and he would call me if he needed me.

The media interviewed Bo and talked with the bereaved parents. Bo and the parents were filmed signing the application for reparations. In spite of Bo's orders, I made my way to the supply room, which was not far from his staged performance. As I approached the door, I saw the bereaved parents about to leave the Court. As they were leaving, many people were gathered in the hallway by the exit door of the Court and it looked as if the cameras were still rolling. Bo suddenly made a transparent attempt at a compassionate statement and embraced the murdered child's mother as though he was concerned. If she knew Bo like I knew Bo, she would be able to see right through his game. He was so dramatic. He saw me looking, but he pretended not to. Afterwards, he called me to his office. He wanted to know how I thought he would look on television. Then he asked me if I saw the part when he hugged the mother. He said, "Damn, that's going to look great. I want you to get a blank videotape and record it and bring it into the office tomorrow." And just like an enslaved servant, that night I videotaped the news and brought it in the next day, just as he demanded.

Journal Entry XIV

Bo made it mandatory to have a staff meeting every morning

at 8:30 a.m. It was unheard of to be late. If so, you would catch hell and be talked about during your absence. In our daily morning staff meetings, Bo would demonstrate his illusive powers and stroke his ego by ordering people around and creating a measure or two of humiliation at will. Everyday, there were the same five or six administrative staff members in these meetings; Bo, Robert, Lillian, Lindsey, Tim, the fiscal officer and myself. Sometimes, Clerk Derfth or Jack, an attorney for the Court, would pop in.

On one particular morning, Bo decided to grace us with one of his sexist jokes. He said, "I heard that the bigger the boobs, the dumber the broad." He paused, made eye contact with the breast of the females in the meeting, smirked, and said, "That means Carson, Brewster and Watson should be real smart." We were the only females present. Everybody laughed, except for me, Robert, and Tim. I didn't find it humorous at all and thought that it was very unprofessional for a director to talk like that to his staff. Perhaps the others laughed because it was in their best interest to laugh. If Bo told a joke, Bo expected everybody who worked for him to laugh. And they did, just like mindless puppets.

Bo totally abused his power and authority as Director of the Victims of Crime Compensation Program. The Clerk, was an older, white male attorney and a former military man. It appeared that he, too, was afraid of Bo. His salt and pepper hair was always neatly parted and combed to the side revealing his meticulous appearance and demeanor. Many lines of maturity were etched in his square shaped face and if you looked close, you could see the sun's signature on his skin. There were faint traces of sun spots on his fair skin. One would guess that he enjoyed plenty of outdoor activities. Perhaps tennis or swimming.

In listening to the Clerk's conversations, I got the impression that he was well read and well traveled. He stood about 5 '11"and for a man his age, he appeared to be in good physical condition. I was told that he was a former pilot and command officer in the United States Air Force and possessed a Juris Doctorate. One would be tempted to think of him as an authoritative figure. But Bo revealed that Clerk Derfthe had no respect or authority in the Court of Claims. Bo outwardly calls the Clerk, "Spuds". His name is Mike Derfthe. Bo said that they were both appointed by the Supreme Court Justice Douglas J. Morton. Bo's evil dictatorial persona swallowed and overshadowed Clerk Derfthe's so called authority. Bo ate it up, spit it out, and stomped on it. And sadly enough, the Clerk let it happen.

"Stay away from Mike! Don't talk, interact or even smile at him," Bo commanded me, "Or you'll be looking for another job." Somehow, Bo found a way to torture me everyday.

Journal Entry XV

Today my phone rang. It was Bo. He ordered me to come to his office. I hated how I had to be at his beck and call. He gives me orders just because he can. Sometimes, he will call me to his office and upon entering, he will undress me with his lustful eyes, tell me to leave and get back to work, and I will leave out feeling as though I have been raped. I was very angry with myself for allowing this to happen over and over and because I didn't have anywhere to turn for help. It's a very difficult thing to explain this kind of bondage and why I participate in enslaving myself to Bo. The Supreme Court Justice, the silent Clerk of Courts, and a Monster Director, being permitted to do whatever he wants... all three, powerful men. More powerful than I?

This particular time, Bo called me to his office, visually undressed me and told me to close the door and have a seat. My heart was beating with fear, deep and hard. I felt that Bo had the Court so afraid of him that if he chose to rape me in his office and I cried for help nobody would come. Except Robert. But he wasn't around. I couldn't concentrate when I was alone with Bo. He made me nervous and I dreaded the day he would make full sexual advances towards me. What will I do? I hated Bo for making my days so full of hell and I hated myself for allowing him to control me. I felt trapped, betrayed and ashamed.

After I sat down, he just stared for almost two long penetrating, minutes. Then he began to burp out his commands. "Patricia, this morning, you gave me a letter to review when "Spuds" was in my presence. Don't ever do that again, he yelled, as he banged on his dusty-topped desk with his fist of fury. In between banging, he would point his long finger in my face. "The letter was no big deal," he continued to growl, "But what I do is none of Mike's business. If he's around when you hand me something, he may give me his stupid two-cent suggestions and fuck everything up. Mike is a fuck-up! You do know that, don't you? That's why I runs this Court! That's why I call him *Spuds.* He's an ass hole! And I don't want to see you or hear tell of you talking to him about any project that I assign you. Understand! All you better ever do or say is hi and bye to the ass hole, 'cause I don't have time to clean up after his mess. If I catch you doing otherwise, you're fired! Is that clear!?"

"Yes, Sir, Boss." By then I had learned to respond to Bo in that manner. "Yes, sir, boss," seems to calm the beast in him down. If I don't say it, he'll badger me until I do. I can't help feeling as if I'm on a cotton plantation taking orders from my slave master.

Then in an most eerie manner, his voice calmed down and he walked toward me, touched me on my shoulders and leered at my breast and said, "Go on, get out of here and get back to work. By the way, that blue silk dress looks mighty good on you. Is it new? "Yes Sir, Boss," I said in the most cold, non-emotional way I could get away with. Then he plopped his big square rusty ass back on his throne. In his mind, he definitely was KING. In my mind, I certainly felt like his servant...

(Thoughts)

None of your damned business you big black, ugly, mental, bastard. And if you don't stop starring at me I'm going to kick your ass. And the next time you touch me, I'm going to kick your balls to hell where they belong.

Instead, I silently got up and walked toward the door. Just before I turned the door knob to leave, Bo called my name. I cringed and stopped my actions midstream. I froze. He said my name again with a commanding and threatening tone. I felt a knot well up in my throat but somehow, I managed to turn around. I turned around, took one step and my breast and face crashed dead into his Humpty-Dumpty shaped torso. How he got up from behind his desk and managed to get so close to me and stop my forward motion, was spooky and unreal. One second he was sitting behind his desk and the next second he had me blocked between his body and the door.

I was so close to him that I smelled cigarette smoke on his breath, and his body musk. I could feel and hear his evil heart beat. It sounded so loud I was almost unaware that my own heart was beating rapidly with fear. My emotions felt far removed from my body. My heart felt as if it were a million miles apart from my chest. I stood there like a mannequin, frozen in time. He wrapped his elongated, octopus arms around my entire petite body and like a captured squirrel, I was afraid to move. He rubbed my butt and backside and held the side of my head in place against his rib cage and softly whispered, "You're doing a great job, Patricia. I've got big plans for you. You just need to loosen up a bit, relax and act right, okay?" Then he released his ape-like grip, and I turned and walked out, dazed and helpless. I felt totally invaded. I went to the restroom and cried. I cried because I felt powerless and there was nowhere for me to go for help. There was no EEO Officer in this Court and Bo served as my director and supervisor. I was truly all alone.

Journal Entry XVI

Bo had the kind of touch that penetrated your clothing and chilled your bones and his spirit exuded evil. I was not used to being embraced by a demon-possessed person, and it gave me chills and created nausea and imbalance in my spirit. I didn't quite know how to protect myself from his evil.

Momma and Daddy always taught me that prayer protects, prepares, provides and prevents. After what Bo did to me yesterday, I knew I was not dealing with flesh and bone, but something spiritually evil. Darkness against the light. My prayers have to be answered soon. God's word has to come through. I feel like I'm losing hope and vision... then I shall surely perish. Please Lord....

I had no idea what God was preparing me for. All I know is that after Bo hugged me and chilled my spirit, I was deeply compelled to pray, fast, read the word, and wait upon the Lord.

I really wanted to talk to my Pastor, Dr. Washington, about Bo. He's a very concerned pastor who is strong in spirit, and anchored in the word. But I couldn't make myself confide my troubles in him. Part of me felt ashamed. I used the excuse that the pastor is too busy addressing needs of other member and I didn't want to burden him. Jeff told him about it though. And he kept us in prayer. I made it a requirement to be at church on Sundays so I could stay spiritually balanced. Mt. Hermon has mighty prayer warriors and I'd go up for prayer every time it was offered.

I prayed for God to give me strength and words powerful enough to put Bo in his place and the authority to make him leave me alone. The words never came. My tongue remained tied. I was never able to successfully defend myself against this evil man. All I had were tears of anger and frustration. I thought I was going to lose my mind.

Almost every morning, I would arrive at work around 7:30 and I would read my Bible, pray and meditate in my office cubicle, asking God to give me strength to make it through the day without letting Bo get me down.

Although I know prayers do not go unheard or unanswered, I felt nor saw no deliverance from this maniac. Finally, I to called Momma and Daddy and ask them to pray for me. I have been delivered and protected from evil many things because of their prayers. I know I am wrapped up and protected by the prayers of my elders. Now I must call upon their strength. I was too weak and I needed the help of *prayer warriors*.

All I can say now is God have mercy on your soul, Bo Gilyard. God's judgement and vengeance is like none other. When my momma and daddy puts you on the altar in prayer, they leave you there, and before it is all said and done, you'll know without a doubt that God is dealing with you. And when God whips your butt, you'll know it's kicked. It's a butt whippin' that can't be stopped by anybody or anything except through the true repentance of your heart.

Daddy and Momma came down to Columbus to see how I was doing. Daddy, bless his heart, hates to see any of his baby girls get mistreated and he was anxious to get with Bo man to man. Momma and Daddy comforted me in their own way and suggested that I fast and pray and be very careful not to shut family and friends out. Momma said I must find my joyful moments among loved ones. They wanted me to come home to visit them more often. But I knew I couldn't without risking my job. But I'm going to take a day off and do it anyway. Forget Bo. Besides, he's not treating me any better.

Journal Entry XVII

I am under so much stress. I feel God has forsaken me. Today, when I was visiting my parents in Oberlin, sharing with them the latest incident regarding Bo, I got very nauseous and my head started spinning around in circles as if I were on a non-stop merry-go-round. My head was spinning out of control and I was forced to drop to the floor. The only escape I had was in closing my eyes, and laying my head in Momma's lap and staying perfectly still. She placed her prayerful hands on my head and the assurance of her touch calmed me. But even with her efforts of comfort, I saw visions of that hideous grin on Bo's face and heard his cursed voice of abuse echoing in my ear. In the background, I could hear somebody dialing numbers on the rotary telephone. Somebody was calling my doctor. He wanted to examine me as soon as possible. My niece, Stephanie, and nephew, Malik, were in Oberlin with me and they were able to drive me back to Columbus, straight to my doctor's office. All I could do was lay out in the back seat of my car and cry silent tears with my eyes shut. No matter how hard I tried to hold back the flood of my anguish, my tears seeped through the slits of my heavy latent eyes.

During the entire 2-hour drive, I cried tears of anguish and on occasion, I heard myself moaning, and groaning. As stupid as it may seem, I was haunted by the thought of not being able to work the next day. I was afraid of the possibility of Bo getting angry. He invades my every thought with evil and sexual connotations. He was haunting me, even as I lay dying.

We arrived safely to the doctor's office. While being examined by my doctor, I wanted so much to tell him about my sexual harassment problems at work. At the same time, I was concentrating so much on being strong and holding back tears that I thought my brain was going to explode. Why can't I cry now that I'm here? Why can't I release everything. I wanted to confess my weakness right there in his office. For some reason, I thought I would be instantly healed if I did. But the protective feminine side of me was stronger and would not let me. My pink rationale felt that a

45

man could not possibly understand or begin to relate to the internal pain I felt. The fragmentation I was experiencing and the type of healing I sought could not possibly come from a man. And the thought of confiding in a White man about a problem I was having with a Black man didn't appeal to my cultural core either. My lips would not part nor could I cry for the help I so desperately needed. My doctor must have noticed that I was depressed or had something on my mind because he asked me if everything was going alright in my life? I said, "Yes, for the most part." I was hoping that he could see right through my words and read my mind. I was hoping he would ask me more question, but he didn't. The little scared child inside of me was crying out loud, and he didn't hear her, so he didn't know to ask -- and I never got to say how much I was hurting.

I was diagnosed as having vertigo. My equilibrium was out of whack and that made me feel extremely dizzy every time I stood up or looked around at moving objects. My doctor asked me what other symptoms I was experiencing. I told him that I kept a hollow-like feeling in the pit of my stomach most of the time. Other times, I had severe diarrhea. When standing up, I felt like I had to vomit, and every time I opened my eyes, I felt a strong spinning sensation. I couldn't walk a straight line. I was unable to stand or walk without leaning on someone or being held up by a wall.

He said that this condition could be triggered by a cold or stress. I didn't have a cold at all. I knew it was from my stressful and hostile work environment with Bo. I was told there was no particular cure for this ailment. My doctors orders were bed rest for a week and to take some type of medication to minimize my symptoms of nausea and dizziness. I was instructed not to drive because this illness distorted my perception of true direction. I could actually be crossing the center line while driving because my brain would be signaling that I was driving straight when I would be driving at an angle, or something weird like that. My driving would create a serious hazard for all other drivers, too.

Just think, I can't walk, read, stand, drive, or look at my loved ones without feeling deeply ill, but for some insane reason, I was still trying to figure out how Bo was going to react to me not coming to work.

Bo has no compassion. His abuse and evilness had finally got to me. I felt totally helpless. This bastard finally broke me. I was so obsessed with doing a good job and trying to handle his sexual abuse by myself that my whole internal being was rendered "out of balance". Can you imagine a soul or a universe out of balance? Confusion, violence, disorder and finally, destruction! *"Oh Lord, my strength, my redeemer, please help me!"*

Journal Entry XVIII

As I lay here at home in bed with my eyes closed, I'm still haunted by Bo's anticipated reaction. I practiced over and over again in my mind how I was going to explain things to him. I even fantasized that when I explained my illness to him, He would be understanding and concerned. What a joke! Like a hypnotized fool, I went back to work, earlier than my doctor recommended. Bo met me in the hallway and instantly he started messing with me. He started with fast rocking motions from side to side to make me dizzy. He kept doing it until he saw me stumble to the wall. Then he whined an insidious laugh. Oh, God, this man is so very mental. Why on earth are you allowing this fool to live and ruin other people? Bo's constant, rapid movements made my head swell like an inner tube and swim like a fish. My stomach began to churn and well up like I had to vomit. I began to heave over and over, but nothing came up. Oh how I wished I could have vomited all over his face. I just stood with my head hung down, one arm wrapped around stomach and the other arm holding onto the wall -- like a black yard ornament holding a lamp. Then a most frightening thought entered my mind. Who told him I had vertigo?

Journal Entry XIX

This indeed would be a challenging day. Bo ordered me to chauffeur him to Cleveland so he could give a speech. The day had been long and my body was tired. I knew this was going to be a trying time for me. I was hoping that Bo would not speak to me at all during the entire drive. But wishful thinking was not powerful enough to cease the derogatory flow of comments he needed to say to make himself feel big.

Cleveland was going to be about a three and a half hour

drive from where we were. While I played chauffeur, Bo made conversation. Then he asked my opinion on a few issues. I've learned to respond to him by agreeing with everything he says. Bo seeks your opinion, then he dares you to disagree with him. If you disagree, he responds with his demonic raft of cursing, badgering, and staring at you in hopes of intimidating you. And after a while, you learn to deal with his madness by agreeing with him outwardly and inwardly thinking, "Hell no!" So when he asked me if his speech was more exciting than the other speakers. I just said, "Yes."

(Thoughts)

Hell no, it wasn't. But whether it was or not, was of no interest to me; I'm focused on getting to our destination and getting out of the car with this beast.

Then Bo reached over and patted me on my upper thigh and said, "You did a good job today, Patricia, good job." I flinched. Bo's touch was more than a touch of flesh to flesh. It invaded my personal space and his touch was unwanted by me. When he touched me it felt like his touch shattered my aura and turned it a cold, deep shade of gray. His spirit exuded evil vibes and felt like the tips of his fingers were tainted with a negative charge that pierced my flesh and cooled my soul like ice. I hated him touching me at will.

When he patted my thigh, I said nothing. There was at least two full minutes of silence after he touched me. This was one of those touches that Momma use to tell me about when I was a little girl. The unwanted, forbidden touch from a stranger and its hidden danger was happening now. Momma said to never keep it a secret when someone touches me on my private place or wanted me to touch them on their private place.

I never had to tell Momma that I had been touched like that as a child. Now as an adult woman, I know what she meant. Bo's touch had crossed the boundaries that Momma warned me about. But Momma was no where around and me and Momma never got a chance to talk about what I should do if a stranger touched me on my private place. I couldn't run and tell. I just kept silent. All I knew to do was to keep silent. For one brief moment though, I think Bo felt uncertain of his effect on me.

When we were about 45 miles from Cleveland, Bo yawned loud enough to annoyingly break the silence. He told me he was closing his eyes for a while and take a nap. I just said, "Ok, that sounds like a good idea. I'll wake you up when we get to the exit." How great it would be if I could just close my eyes and wake up at home with my family.

As Bo lay back with his eyes closed, I glanced over at him. My friend Patty always said, "Every shut eye ain't sleep." I knew Bo wasn't really sleep, but even as he pretended, he had frown lines etched around his mouth and engraved across his forehead. His round bald head leaned backwards forcing the corners of his mouth to droop. His pointed ears pertruded from his bald head as if they were trying to take up wings and fly. Perhaps they knew they could better serve their purpose on someone else head. On Bo's head they were only allowed to function on the level of a hairless jackass. I could feel his brain plotting as he pretended to sleep.

My thoughts kept roaming. I was thinking how Bo enjoyed compliments about his suits and the expensive shirts and ties he wore. He prided himself on being a conscientious dresser. He wanted so much to be a "big shot". He would give his dry cleaner receipts to Robert so that Robert could pick his clothes up from the cleaners. He took pleasure in passing Robert his dry cleaner's receipts in front of other people too. It made Robert feel like a flunky and made Bo feel in charge. Bo wanted people to wait on him hand and foot, i.e. carrying his brief case, opening the door for him, and chauffeuring him around. He made some of us run personal errands for him, too.

Robert was Bo's victim just like I was. But Bo only went so far with Robert. Probably because Robert knew too much about Bo's bad ethics, work habits, prior marriages, girlfriends and obsession with pornography. Robert told me about Bo's questionable political activities and misuse of overnight hotel accommodations while on state business to meet women. He said it made him feel uncomfortable to even be around when Bo decided to act like that.

Bo made many of us work on James Litchovich's campaign in his quest for governorship. If Litchovich only knew how Bo broke rules and laws on behalf of the gubernatorial election campaign, he would flip!

I started humming, the Lord's Prayer in hopes of keeping myself focused and protected. My humming got louder and louder. I was trying to take my mind off of *Big, Bad, Bo.* I knew he wasn't really asleep. After about 15 minutes, he pretended to wake up with aggravated abruptness while I was humming the last of the Lord's Prayer, *...but deliver us from evil*, and in a raspy voice he said, "Are we in Cleveland yet?!"

Before I could answer, Bo continued talking. I thought of the song *"Talking Loud and Saying Nothing"*, as I half listened to him. I concentrated on the mileage count down to the exit much like an astronaut counting down to landing.

I was very tired and looked forward to getting to my hotel room and relaxing. My stomach was growling since I hadn't eaten dinner. I think he heard my stomach or either his felt empty too. Bo suggested that we check into our hotel rooms, freshen up a bit and then go out to dinner.

Upon arrival at the hotel, we approached the hotel clerk to check-in. Bo had already told me that I would be in the room reserved for Robert. Now he wants me to sign the hotel register as Robert. I did sign Robert's name but I added my initials to indicate that it was me and not Robert, who was the occupant.

Of all the rooms I could have received, the clerk or Bo arranged for our rooms to be side by side. Lord, I hope our rooms do not have connecting doors. As I put my key in my door, Bo said,

"Call me, Patricia, when you are ready to go to dinner. Don't take too long because restaurants are about to close." I said, "Okay," entered my room and quickly closed my door. Hurriedly, I splashed some water on my face, washed my hands, then called Bo and said, "I'll meet you in the hallway in two minutes." I didn't even want him to get a glimpse of the inside of my room.

We went to a restaurant a few blocks from the hotel. There were only a few people in the restaurant. We placed our order and waited on our food. While waiting, Bo began talking about his marriage. He asked how Jeff and I got along. I told him, "Jeff and I have lots of challenges like any married couple, but we're happy. We've had close calls but we continue to work hard to make our marriage a good marriage. And like all relationships, you have to be positive, seek solutions and make an effort to support each other." It sounded like a short motivational speech that was void of motivation. But I dared not give out too much enthusiasm to Bo about my happiness!

As a trainer and motivational speaker, people find it easy to confide in me about their personal and professional problems. But Bo's conversation seemed to be heading in a direction that was full of sexual innuendoes and since he's so full of bulls..t, I was very careful to take the posture of just listening without moving my body or showing any facial expressions. I didn't shake my head in agreement or disagreement. I placed my hands under the table and stared straight ahead and tried to disappear.

But Bo kept talking about some phobia he claimed he had. It sounded more like a sexual fantasy rather than a phobia. I was forced to listen with great inner agitation as he told me how he could not drive over bridges or on long winding roads. "If I do, the road appears to move and become distorted and can cause me to wreck," he claimed. I really didn't understand what he was talking about and truly didn't care. I couldn't help but wonder how he managed to get home everyday since he has to drive over a bridge in order to get there. This man is so full of bull it ain't funny!

Anyway, Bo continued, "The doctor gave me medication to help control my phobia. But my medication made me impotent, and I couldn't get a "hard-on". I hadn't had a hard-on in a long time and it caused a strain on my marriage. I misplaced my frustrations on the job and worked long hours as a means to escape and relieve some of my pressure. One day I stopped taking the medication. Not long after that I discovered that I was able to get a "hard on". Now my sex drive is back. I'm pissed off with my doctor for not telling me that impotence was a side effect of the medicine. I cursed his ass out too, but at the same time I'm relieved to find out that I can get a hard dick," he chuckled.

Here I am sitting here listening to all of this inappropriate crap from my boss's mouth. I felt embarrassed, humiliated, uncomfortable, frightened, and pissed all at the same time about this entire conversation. I don't give a damn about Bo's penis! Uck! It's enough to make you throw up. I'm out here in a strange place all alone with a maniac that has rediscovered his dick. All I could think of is who care's about this fool's dick. I ain't the one to be happy for you fool. Tell you wife. The only reason the conversation was brought to an end is because the restaurant was getting ready to close and they needed us to leave so that they could finish closing.

When we got back to the hotel, Bo walked me to my door and I said good night. I put my key in the door and he said, "Wait a minute Patricia, let's talk about tomorrow." I sighed and stood still. We had already talked about tomorrow in the car. He was just stalling for time. I think he hoped that I would open my door and ask him to come on in. Instead, I pulled my door back shut and stood there in the hallway. I waited for him to tell me what else he felt I needed to know about tomorrow. I looked at my watch, it was getting pretty late!

He didn't say much of anything about tomorrow. Instead, he started asking about my marriage again. He asked, "Were you married when I first met you? I bet Jeff really enjoys being married to you, huh?" He kept staring at me. His eyes were roving up and down the full length of my body. I tried hard not to respond one way or the other. I just stood there thinking, please, Lord, don't let this man touch me. It's difficult to tell what one word can set an unstable mind off, so I remained unresponsive to his questions about my personal life and while he was telling me how sensuous I was and how he would like to have me for himself. After about 20 minutes of silence and cold shoulder, I said, "Well Bo, if there is nothing else, good night. I have not had an opportunity to call my husband and he expects me to call him tonight and tell him about my trip. I'll talk with you in the morning." With that, I turned, unlocked my door, entered quickly, and shut the door in his face. I left him standing in the hallway,"*holding his dick"* as they say.

I checked and rechecked my door to ensure that it was locked. I placed a chair under the door knob for added security. This made me feel a little safer from Bo. I called my husband and told him I felt uncomfortable around Bo. I didn't go into a lot of details. I could tell that Jeff was concerned. He said he was coming to Cleveland. I said, "No honey, I'm just tired. I'll be home tomorrow. I'll be ok. Good night, and pray for us, and remember I love you. Bye."

The next morning, Bo and I went to breakfast. He read the newspaper and talked while we were waiting to be served. Then, out of the blue, he began telling me sexual jokes. He said, "Patricia, want to hear something funny?" Before I could answer, he started into it.....

There was a guy named Long Dick Willie. His dick was 10 feet long and his dick scared women away. He tried women on the east and west coast and women would always run from his big dick. One day out of frustration, Long Dick Willie cried and complained to his best friend. His friend arranged for him to meet a woman who could take every inch of his dick. He met the woman and they began to fuck. Willie was afraid she would not be able to handle his long dick so he eased it in her slowly. Much to his surprise, she kept saying more, more, more. Long Dicked Willie had finally met the perfect pussy and he asked her how does it feel. She responded. (At this point, Bo quickly stuck his tongue in and out to indicate that Long Dick Willie's penis had come up through her throat and was moving in and out of her mouth).

Then Bo, started laughing, leaned forward, and slid right into the next sick joke.

.... This fellow suspected that his wife was cheating on him so he hired a hit man to follow her and catch her in the act. The hit man was instructed to shoot his wife in the middle of the head and to shoot his wife's lover in the ball. The hit man said, "Fine, but I charge $1,000 for each bullet I have to use." They agreed upon $2,000. The husband and the hit man followed the wife and her lover to a hotel and they watched them enter the room together. They were so anxious to start fucking that they forgot to close the window blinds so the hit man could see them very well through the telescope on his rifle. The hit man began to describe to the husband what they were doing. He said they were kissing and feeling all over one another and he explained how they fell onto the bed. The husband shouted out, "What are you waiting for, shoot 'em!" The hit man said, just be patient, if you just wait a minute, she's going down one him, to give

57

him a blow job. Then, I can get you two for the price of one bullet."

Bo just kept rolling right along with his demonic laughing and telling jokes. He's sick! Who can I tell about this powerful man? If I only had a tape recorder. He acted like a eight year old kid at Christmas time, who was excited about his first bicycle. "How about this one," he continued with gleam in his eyes.

"There was a nerd who could never get a date to go to bed with him because every time he would take off his clothes the women would laugh at him because his dick was so tiny. On New Years Eve he was all by himself in a hotel room. He thought about getting laid and began to make a wish. His wish was so sincere that a genie appeared and said he would grant the nerd one wish. Since the nerd never had sex, he really, really wanted to have sex. He thought that if he had a penis like a "nigger", women would have sex with him. So he said, "I wish I was 'hung like a nigger'." The genie said, "Your wish is my command," and disappeared. The nerd was quite anxious for his change to come. He waited and waited and kept looking at his dick, but he saw no change. Finally, he heard a knock at the door. He opened the door and saw three large men with white cone-shaped hoods on their heads. Holding a noose, they asked, "Are you the one who wanted to be hung like a nigger?"

Bo laughed so hard behind that one, I thought he was going

to fall out of his chair. Wished he had of. We ate and left for the conference.

I didn't know many people there, but I knew my cousin Curtis was scheduled to be there and I kept checking at NABCJ's registration desk and leaving messages for him. But I never made contact with him. I wanted to tell him about Bo and get him to make Bo back off of me.

Bo gave his speech as scheduled. And as usual, at the end of his speech, he tried to hug every female in the room that would let him, while I cleaned up and packed up our supplies. Just out of curiosity, I glanced at his left hand and just as I predicted, Bo had removed his wedding band and slipped it in his pocket. Bo did that almost every time he'd have a speaking engagement. I guess he wanted women to think he was available. It was so noticeable though because it left a light spot on his ring-finger where his wedding band was suppose to be. I was happy that the conference ended and that I was headed home. I never did find my cousin Curtis.

Bo was talkative on the way home, but his attitude was different and he appeared to be overly anxious to get back to the office. We had not eaten lunch. Bo said that he did not want to stop and get anything to eat because he wanted to get back to the office before Spuds fucked things up. So, of course, I had to starve to accommodate his paranoid thoughts. He called the office from the car phone to check up on everything. Then, out of the blue, Bo asked me to pull over and let him drive. He said I was driving too slow. I was going the speed limit. I immediately pulled over and he drove. He drove for about 10 or 12 miles, and he kept nervously looking in the rear view mirror. He asked me if a car he saw way in back of us was a highway patrolman. I looked back to see what he was talking about and I couldn't believe that he wanted me to tell him whether or not the highway patrol was behind us. The car he was talking about was so far away, it looked like a dot. He continued driving. As the car behind us got closer, Bo's hands started jerking at the steering wheel and made the car swerve. He claimed that his phobia was making him sick and that he needed to exit quickly and let me drive. But seconds before the next exit, the car that was behind us, passed us. Bo was right, it was the State Highway Patrol. He must have the eyes of an eagle. When the trooper passed us, Bo's hands started shaking harder. This fool is probably wanted for something. Maybe he doesn't have a license. If he doesn't have a license, why is he in permanent possession of a state released vehicle? Anyway, he was sure scaring the heck out of me. I thought he was getting ready to convulse under the wheel.

When we arrived back in the office, I told Robert what happened during my trip to Cleveland and how Bo tried over and over to hit on me. I told Robert about Bo telling me all kinds of sexual jokes. While Robert and I were talking, our conversation was interrupted with a telephone ring. It was Bo. He said he wanted to see me in his office right away. I went. He asked me to step in and close the door. I did. Bo was writing something. He never lifted his pen from the paper nor did he lift his head to visually acknowledge my presence. He just said,"Patricia, you won't accompany me out of town anymore." "What?" I asked. Bo repeated himself. "Why?" I said with a suspicious tone. Bo lifted his head in slow motion, and with well aimed piercing eyes, he looked at me and said, "Simple, you should stay home and take care of your wifely duties with Jeff." Then he looked back down at his paper to finish writing with one hand while he motioned with his other hand in a go-on-get-out-of-here gesture. Like he was shoeing a fly. I left.

Bo was just pissed off because he couldn't sex me when we were in Cleveland. In his mind, it was a waste of time to allow me to accompany him on business trips if there was no pleasure involved. Which is perfectly fine with me. I knew this wouldn't be the end of it though. I didn't know how far this man was going to take this whole thing but because he's vindictive I shuttered at how he would retaliate. My guts told me that my life on the job was going to get worse. And it did.

Journal Entry   XX

Today, Bo called me into his office and asked me for a brief update of my activities. I already conveyed my activities to him this morning in our mandatory staff meetings. But I gladly repeated my activities to him. As usual, he interrupted me before I could finish and in a soft growl, said, "Mrs. Carson, I am assigning you a project.

It's been underway for close to two years prior to your employment at the Court. This project had been previously assigned to other staff here along with volunteer staff members of other agencies. Why don't you knock the dust off of it and get it done. It's very tedious and painstaking," and almost with laughter in his throat, he continued, "But I'm certain you're the right person to get the job done. I want a status report on my desk, outlining exactly what has been done, and what has not been done on this project so that we can get this thing accessed and finished. You're to identify every community service organization in the state of Ohio, in all 88 counties and determine whether or not these agencies still exist. If so, what community services they provide, who they service and who the current contact person is. On top of that I want current addresses, telephone numbers, and other relevant information that is required to put together an efficient statewide community service directory. It that clear?" With a vertical wave of his hand, he shooed me away, saying, "Now, get out of here and get back to work!

PROJECT REVENGE had begun. He's getting his revenge. Rumor was that this project had been passed around like a hot potato. Prior to my coming to work in this court, a whole team of people worked on it and failed to complete the job. It was considered grunt or dirty work. Bo was more than happy to do me the honors. When all the paperwork for PROJECT REVENGE was placed on my desk, it looked so overwhelming that my eyes started to water. I could feel my tear ducts filling up. He was getting his revenge for my rejection and I knew it. The community service organizations for all 88 counties in Ohio amounted to piles and piles of computer print out sheets and stacks of files with what looked like hundreds and hundreds of listed service agencies. I had to review these print outs, sheet by sheet, item by item, and then compare that information with data that had been entered months ago into a computer program by individuals who had started this project before. Bo felt that I could handle it all alone and he demanded that I get him the results of my status report on his desk quick and in a hurry. He made it perfectly clear that he expected me to keep up with my other duties as well.

My eyes, and back were in constant pain for weeks. But I had to keep going. I couldn't afford to give him an excuse to say I was not producing timely and quality work. I'm a very organized and creative person. With this project, I had to pull forth all my talents. I developed a color coded system to separate the data he required. I found myself, humming old spiritual songs to keep me uplifted. At the same time, I couldn't help but wonder how many other women, past and present, have endured worse treatment than I, some from sun up to sun down, with no sign of relief, just for a paycheck. Some for no pay at all...

Just say no to drugs and it becomes a step in the ladder of success. Just say no to sex, and your ladder suddenly breaks into a million pieces and soon you're left dangling by a splinter of wood and labeled as a disgruntled employee.

Everyday, I prayed the prayer of God's revenge on Bo's head just as the Psalmist did. I know within my heart, that God is going to make him feel the pain he creates and pay him back for his evil ways. I just wished it would happen now. I was counting down the days for Bo to get his appointment to the governor's cabinet he's always bragging about.

If I could just keep the faith. If I could just hold out, in God's own time, my change will come.

My sisters Corgie, Monica, and Toni and my friend Marie helped me tremendously. One day Marie came downtown and had lunch with me. We talked about positive things. She was catching hell of a different kind on her job. But we were never too overburdened to check on one other every now and then and see how each was holding out. Marie and I have a long history together. We have supported one another through our years of poverty. At that time, she had two daughters and I had two sons and we were both on public assistance living in a Section 8 Housing community.

There were four of us Afrikan American sisters who lived in the same housing development. We were all divorced single parents, in college, trying to change our future. Betty, Carla, Marie, and me. We shared everything. We had to in order to survive. Betty cooked the best navy beans I've ever tasted. We ate beans at Betty's at least once a week. Her son Courtney was a classmate and friend with my two sons, Dorian and Derrick. Marie refused to eat a single bean no matter how good I said they were. She said she had too many beans from her childhood days in Harlem. She swore she was allergic. But Marie could do wonders with chicken.

Carla and I weren't much of a cook but Carla had the most uncanning ability to always see the bright side of life. She taught us how not to sweat the small stuff. To her it was all small stuff. We watched one anthers back and developed a spiritual sisterhood and kept one another going.

I had a used car with a loud muffler. Sometimes, I was the designated driver on food stamp day. This was the longest day of the month. Standing in those long lines was an humiliating experience for us but we would use that time to plan a better future. It was difficult to stay focused on positive thoughts with so many negative things coming at you. But we managed.

One day my car got repossessed. I only owed $600 more dollars on it. I cried for two days. Then I had to wipe my face and focus on surviving. These were the times I wondered how in the world my sons father could neglect them by showing no interest in their well-being. He never knew if they had boots, coats, or gloves in the winter time. He never asked. But between my parents, Grand daddy Coy and Momma Leon, Aunt Vern, Charity Newsies, and thrift shops, we did alright.

Carla could find the best spots in town to get second hand clothes. We would go to the best thrift shops in the suburbs. They sold a lot of designer labels. We could take someone elses' give-a-ways, and turn them into outfits that would make *Henri Bendel* take notice. We always looked like we had money in our pockets and wouldn't have a dime. Those were the days.

Marie and I were the only two that managed to graduate from college. But all of us promised that we would always be there for one another no matter what the future brought. Both of us landed the state government jobs we dreamed of while we stood in the food stamp lines. Now, neither of us knew why we had that dream in the first place.

Years after the realized dream, over lunch, Marie is offering to kick my supervisor's butt for me. We both knew that wasn't going to happen, but the thought sounded good and she made me laugh. She said, "You take one leg and I'll take the other and together, we'll whip his a..." Her concern was genuine and we parted with our sisterly embrace. Marie squeezed me so hard I thought she was trying to squeeze the pain out of me. It didn't work, but I felt the power of her spirituality. We both knew in due time, Bo was going to get his.

Journal Entry XXI

I can't wait for Bo to leave so I won't have to be concerned with sexual harassment. I'll have better opportunities and I'll be able to enjoy my job and duties. Bo has a nasty way of turning good into bad. But God will get him. His dog day is a comin'!

Journal Entry   XXII

Within a few weeks, I provided Bo with the results of PROJECT REVENGE. He said that I did a very good job. He asked me to present my findings in the next staff meeting. I did. My findings cited everything Bo requested. The presentation and attached memo were neat, easy to follow, and comprehensive. Finally, I felt a sigh of relief.

He couldn't wait to give me some more grunt work. Before the day was over, he gave me another project he said he had assigned to Lillian prior to my employment. He wanted me to create an In-house Lending Library. He wanted me to clean off his bookshelves, gather books, journals, and documents of pertinent information throughout the Court for this project. So I gathered books, journals, etc., I typed out book titles, authors, volume number, number of copies on hand, and assigned catalogue numbers.

Once again, for weeks, my desk was covered with what looked like mountains of books and journals. I fought back the tears as I heard the master's whip crackin' in my ear and felt the sting of it's blow. My sister Toni came by unannounced to check up on me. After she left, Bo called me into his office and cursed me out about that. Told me I didn't have time to socialize and that he wants an update of the Lending Library. I was already going at full speed. I didn't have anymore energy to give. I had better get creative and sneak and ask for help from the clerical staff.

I asked the clerical supervisor to help me create a data base. She did and she also lent me the help of one of her data entry clerks to help input the data I had gathered. After a couple of weeks, I was very glad to hand Bo a draft of the In-House Lending Library Catalogue. He okayed it and told me to create room in the already existing Court library and to put up all the books and journals I had cataloged.

On one long, and hard afternoon, while I was working on shelving the books, I had to get down on my hands and knees to put the books in place on the bottom shelf. Out of the blue, Bo came back to the area where I was working. I was so involved with my work, that I was unaware of him approaching me until I felt someone staring at me and I looked up. It was that mental bastard, Bo! He smirked and said, "You look

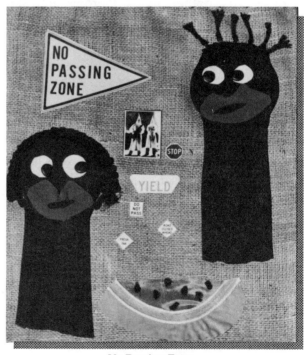

No Passing Zone

good down on your hands and knees, Patricia. Keep up the good work." Then he stepped over me and disappeared around the corner. Bo kept assigning me more and more grunt work and he assigned Robert, my co-worker, less and less work. I felt just like his personal slave. All I could think was, "Lawdy, Lawdy, Lawdy! Bo can't even see for the blindness of his own self-hate. God blessed him to enter doors many Black men are denied. Po' blind Bo --- he thinks its his responsibility to create stumbling blocks for his own people, as if we don't already have more than enough unnecessary obstacles."

Needless to say, Bo was not very happy with the fact that I successfully completed the demeaning projects he gave me. He meant it for bad, - God meant it good. But I now, I'm getting tired.

Journal Entry XXIII

Each day I begin my morning with a prayer for strength and deliverance. I keep a Bible in my desk drawer. The Bible's words of wisdom and promises have become a closer partner. Early one Tuesday morning, I sat in the dark, in my small office space meditating on God's goodness and feeling God's presence. I was too tired to be concerned with my pain, frustrations, or anger. I just sat in silence thinking on God's promises. In that silent moment of surrender, God whispered to me...

"Be still, my child and know that I Am God. I have not forsaken you. My mighty hand shall stretch forth and do

great things through your suffering. Bo Gilyard is a fallen man who thinks he is standing."

Then I read, Exodus 10:1-2 --

...the Lord said unto Moses, Go in unto Pharaoh, for I have hardened his heart, and the heart of his servants, that I might shew these my signs before him; and that thou mayest tell in the ears of they son, and of thy son's son, what things I have wrought in Egypt, and my signs which I have done among them; that ye may know how that I am the Lord.

I knew I was not Moses and there was not an Aaron placed at my side to serve as my communicator. I knew I was not in the land of Egypt and Pharaoh was not my king. But upon reading that passage, I spiritually understood my position and responsibility while on this job.

Bo's heart is hardened. He is not capable of hearing my plea to stop holding me captive to his lascivious whelms. God is going to take care of him through the process of reaping and sowing. The same pain he causes me and others, will be measured out to him. God's infinite wisdom also reminded me not to walk by sight but by faith. At times it may appear as if Bo is standing, but on the spiritual plane he has already fallen. And in due time his fall will manifest itself on the physical plane.

Finally, I saw the light and felt enlightenment and relief. I shared my feelings, revelations and thoughts with a few other people so that when God's word came forth, like a mighty storm, I would have witnesses for God's works, wonders and power. In the meantime, I waited, and waited upon the Lord. It was through knowing that God had already fixed it on the spiritual plane that made my waiting possible and that enabled me to gather inner strength.

Journal Entry XXIV

Hallelujah, Glory, Praises to the Father, Son, and the Holy Ghost, Bo announced today that he had been appointed to the governor's cabinet. Mercy on them! But hallelujah for me! There was much silent joy throughout the Court. Everywhere you could hear whispering about Bo's leaving. Most employees joyously counted down the days for his job change. Even Lindsey, Bo's secretary, was uncertain if she should follow Bo into his new position. Today, Lindsey quietly asked Robert if he was going to follow Bo into his new position. She wasn't quit certain if she should or not.

Seems like everybody in the court rejoiced in their own secret way. It was like a silent Festac Celebration. Although I felt mentally and physically dismembered, I had much joy on the inside. My soul celebrated. I survived the storm! My head is lifted high and there is hope for a better tomorrow. There were a few suggestions of a going away party for Bo. Some contributed money and some didn't. Some said they would attend the party and some said they would not.

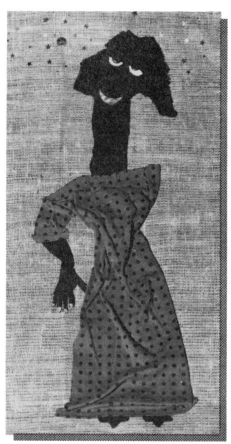

I Survived The Storm

Many mixed feelings surrounded this whole event. The question as to who would take Bo's place as director of the Victims of Crime Compensation Program seemed to get posed the most. Many thought it should be Robert Wyler since he had been part of the Victims Compensation Crime Program almost since its inception. But, Jack Cansinio, the staff attorney, had been attending many closed door meetings with Bo and Mike lately though. Jack's knowledge of the Program appeared to be very minimal compared to that of Robert's. However, politics are politi.

I was just happy Bo was leaving. He didn't give me an evaluation either and at this point, I didn't care. Now I'm no longer subjected to his sexual advances anymore. I did my job, and I outlasted monster Bo! Perhaps under a new administration, I'll be able to work my job under normal, and fair conditions instead of in a hostile environment. No more sexual harassment! Yeah! Inside, I was very happy, happy, happy! I counted every hour of every day waiting for Bo to be gone.

Finally, it was officially announced that Jack Cansinio would be Bo's replacement. I could see that Robert was disappointed. Word was, Bo didn't even consider speaking on behalf of Robert and that he highly recommended Jack. I know Robert must have been disturbed by Bo's lack of loyalty. Not only was Robert very knowledgeable of the Program, Robert is a good employee.

I remember one time Bo made Robert go pick up his teeth (partials) from the dentists. Robert should have thrown them in the Scioto River.

Robert knew Bo was a manipulator and liar. Although Robert was disappointed about Bo's lack of appreciation of his good work, he couldn't have been surprised about Bo promoting Jack over him. He knew Bo.

Journal Entry   XXV

Staff gave Bo his going away party. Hurray! I put in my $3. I looked at it as a cheap ticket to freedom. The monster is finally gone. Our first staff meeting was held with our new director, Jack Cansinio. He wanted each employee to outline their current projects and give him updates on all Victims of Crime Program projects we were working on as individuals. He had very limited knowledge of the program's inner workings. He stated that he would be meeting with each employee to discuss their position, concerns, and just to get a basic feel of everyone's duties.

I was very anxious to be able to speak with Director Cansinio. I was going to tell him about all the sexual harassment difficulties I had experienced while Bo was director and that I was looking forward to working under supervision free of sexual harassment. I drafted a memo, outlining my projects, duties and their status.

After about a week had passed, I noticed that everyone had met with Jack but me. Out of concern, I asked him if he had scheduled me to speak with him yet. He assured me that he had and that my conference would be forthcoming. A couple of days passed and Jack still had not arranged to speak with me, so I inquired with him again. At which time, he said, "Relax, Patricia, I will be getting with you soon." If only he knew, I was more relaxed at work in this job then I've ever been allowed to be, now that big, bad Bo was gone.

Jack, was an attorney for the court. He would often be seen

walking around the court very relaxed and aloof. He seemed to be unbothered about the business of the Court. He reminds me of a life-glider. It was rumored that he taught college during the evenings.

I could see his rather large pitted-face approaching me in the hallways and the minute he was in arms reach, he would extend his hand for a hand shake and softly ask, "What's goin' on?" It was how he greeted me. His hands were warm and soft and reminded me of squeezing a cat.

One time, he approached me in the hallway just outside my cubicle and extended his hand to me. Out of reflex I reached out my hand to reciprocate. Jack grabbed my hand and pulled my hand inward and downward. He pulled me in about 2 inches from his chest and held my hand positioned below his belt. I became furious and pushed back and sarcastically said, "Why don't you just hug me too." Maybe that wasn't the smartest thing to say, but I had flashbacks about Bo's unwanted embrace and touches. I felt that Jack only did that to me because Bo had set up the conditions to make this man feel comfortable enough to disrespect me through the simple gesture of a handshake. I was angry. But still had no where to turn.

During another incident, I was using the copier when I felt someone staring at me. I looked up and saw no one in front or to the sides of me. As I turned my head and looked behind me I saw Jack Cansinio staring in a daze at my behind. I turned and stared

75

back and asked him what was he looking at. I snatched my papers from the copier and continued to stare at him as I walked back to my desk. All I could think of was Bo's sick, lust-filled mind. Bo would tell other male employees that I have the *"nicest ass in the Court."* Not only did he push his illness onto me but his attitude encouraged others to view me as a sex object and not be taken serious as a professional employee. Jack has to know how inappropriate Bo's behavior is. i would hear him sharing things with Robert about Bo. Jack's favorite line about putting up with Bo was, "You've got to go along to get along." And he went along with Bo's program. But then again, I don't think Jack was getting sexually harassed by Bo.

Journal Entry XXVI

On this day, I faced the enormity of the Red Sea alone. Pharaoh (Bo) was in his newly appointed kingdom (position). On the surface, it appeared that things were going quite well for him. But God's words still rang loud in my heart. *Bo Gilyard is a fallen man who thinks he is standing.* How Bo's fall would come about was none of my business. So I thought. Little did I know at that time that God would work through me. Much like David and Goliath.

As I sat at my computer terminal entering data for information and material requests, my telephone rang. I was asked to come up front to the Clerk's Office. I was told that Jack Cansinio and Mike Derfthe wanted to speak with me. I figured it was my first official one on one staff meeting, the one that Jack said he wanted to have with me, so I happily said, "I'll will be right up."

I entered the office and saw Mike and Jack were already sitting. Jack's thick glasses were resting snugly against his large nose. His left fingertips were tapping his right fingertips creating a slow dull rhythm. His facial expression was void of interest and he never said a word. Never said good morning or anything. That seemed strange but not strange enough to prepare me for what I was about to be told.

Mike asked me to shut the door and have a seat. Before I got all the way seated, Mike said, "Based on Bo Gilyard's recommendation, you are being terminated." I could not believe my ears. Mike and Jack both had to know what kind of bastard Bo was! Jack had to have known first hand how Bo treated me and Bo's sexual jokes. Mike told me to pack my personal belongings and leave the premises immediately. I was shocked to the point of nausea.

Once again, I looked at Jack and he looked straight ahead and never said one single word. Through his silence he allowed a grave miscarriage of justice to be imposed upon me. I turned to Mike and asked, "Why?" I had to have and explanation for this madness. All Mike did was gesture his hands in a stop position and repeated himself without emotion, "Based on Bo's recommendation, you are being terminated." He added a little more salt to my open wound and went on to say, "Bo was your supervisor and has personal knowledge of your work performance. I have to go along

77

with his recommendation to terminate you." Again I asked to see my evaluation or something in writing from Bo. Mike stated that he did not have anything. Then he told me that I was to pack my personal belongings and leave the court immediately!

I looked at Jack again and he looked straight ahead like a zombie... *He said nothing.*

(THOUGHT)

I'm still a victim of this Court. A victim, while Bo was here and a victim after he's gone. His servants, are carrying out his biddings. I can't believe this.

As I got up, to leave, Mike reached out to shake my hand and said, "Good luck." Out of reflex, I reached out and shook his wrinkled white hand and said, "Don't worry about me, I'll be alright. (I knew God has already arranged that. God is my source....). I remember thinking though, *"God, are you sure this is how this is suppose to end?"*

I looked again at Jack one last time. He still never said a mumbling word and he never acknowledged me with eye contact. He acted just like a coward that knows he's a coward but had not grown quite accustomed to the truth of his own character.

I could see Bo's face in my mind's eye laughing and pointing his hideous teasing finger at me saying, "I got you!" I walked out of Mike office feeling stripped and cheated. The walk back to my office seemed endless. I was in a total daze. I passed other employees, but they seemed so far away from where I was. Their voices sounded hollow and I felt numb. Everything moved in slow motion, like a scene from the movies. Finally, I arrived back at my computer terminal and the screen message brought me back to reality. My terminal had been shut off with access denied. All the material and information request I did before my nightmare began got torn to shreds and thrown in the garbage. I was sick of being abused. So sick of it. All I felt was hate and contempt for Bo and anger with myself for being so stupid. I see now that Jack had known all along what Bo's plans were for me. My tears began to well up and I fought with all my little might to suppress them. I didn't want these white folk to see me cry. All I remember thinking, was that mental bastard won. He couldn't just leave me alone. He had to reach back and hurt me some more. In that moment, I hated Bo with a great conviction and told God to pure out the raft of revenge for me upon Bo's head. Make him suffer like he has made me suffer. I commanded God to make Bo my footstool. I prayed this prayer from my heart, just like the Psalmist. I prayed that coals of fire would rain on Bo's life for ever and ever until he repents and realizes that he can not keep messing with people lives the way he does.

I felt angry with myself, because if I had of known it was going to come to this end anyway, I would have never begged my husband, my father, my sons, or my friends, not to kick Bo's high-romped, ass like they wanted to. Why had I stopped them! Now, I wish I had the courage and good sense to have cursed him out or kicked him in his balls myself! Now, in the reality of this moment, I felt totally raped. In spite of my broken heart, I knew that God's way was the best way.

I sat at my cubicle not knowing what to do with myself. Robert was on the telephone and I couldn't run straight to him and cry. So I just sat there, fighting back my tears and full of mixed emotions. Bruce, the office manager, kept poking his head in and out of my office space asking me if I needed his help to pack. I kept telling him, "No." Then it hit me, how was I going to get home. I got dropped off at work, like I did everyday. I had no way of getting home. That means I'll have to call Jeff. What's he going to say? Oh God, I just purchased a new living set just three short, happy weeks ago. It was the first living-room outfit that belonged to me. It represented a milestone in my life. For more than fifteen years, I had hand me down furniture or furniture from the goodwill. This set was fresh, new, and beautiful and I was working hard to pay for the joy of owning it. Now how was I to pay? A simple realized dream had suddenly turned into a nightmare!

And, oh my God, what about rent? Groceries? Food? So many thoughts kept rapidly passing through my mind that I began to get dizzy. How will I tell Jeff that I no longer have a job? How will I tell my dad and mom, my sisters and brother? They look up to me for so much. I felt sick. Why didn't Jack say anything? He was the new director now. He could have refused to support Bo's recommendation. But he didn't say a single word. How does he think he would ever make a judge worthy of his robe? In my heart, he never will. And when ever he runs for judge, I will be there to ask him, why he didn't speak up?

I needed to ask Robert if he knew that Bo was going to fire me. And if he did, why didn't he tell me? Finally, I couldn't wait for him to get off of the phone, so I slipped him a note that said *I have an emergency and I need to speak with you right away.*

Robert ended his call and I managed to get the words out of my mouth with teary swollen eyes. I told him that Mike and Jack just fired me. *"What?"* Robert said, as if he had just heard that ghost of Elvis was just spotted roaming the Court. He was very shocked and asked me why. I told him that Mike said it was because Bo recommended that I be terminated. I could see in his eyes and feel in my heart that Robert felt real bad for me. I could tell he was angry and disappointed with the bad news, too.

I told Margie and Celeste. They were secretaries who worked in the same area of the Court as me. Periodically they had heard me complain about how Bo treated me. Margie and Celeste had similar experiences with Bo and from time to time they shared some of those with me. But for a long time, I thought I was the only victim in the court that got abusive treatment from Bo.

It wasn't until I shared it with a few people that I found out that Bo had been creating havoc and sexually harassing other women in the Court for years. No one ever stopped him. Rumor was that he use to openingly date one of his employees and dared his wife to show her face in the court. I know I never saw her visit

81

him at all. I've heard him say that he wished his wife would get run over by a truck. At first I thought he was joking, but he said it too often.

At any rate, I felt like a smashed bug. I cried, and pulled myself together and called Jeff. I just came out straight with it and told him that I had just been fired by Mike Derfthe and Jack Cansinio. I mumbled in a child like voice, and told Jeff that Mike directed me to pack my personal belonging and leave the Court immediately. Jeff asked if I was alright. He could tell by the long pause that I wasn't fighting back my tears. He said, I'll be right there. And as always, he was.

No matter what Bo tried to do to me though, he can't do anything without God's permission. I knew that God was not going to permit Bo to destroy me and that I was placed here in this Court to offer Bo God's redemption. I could feel it in my spirit that this was Bo's last act of blatant abuse of power. Bo's refusal to leave me alone has unleashed the tides of God's raft Bo had set into motion his own destruction.

As I packed, I could hear God's promise being echoed again and again within my mind: *'Bo Gilyard is a fallen man who thinks he is standing... Bo Gilyard is a fallen man, who thinks he is standing'...*

Journal Entry XXVIII

For two weeks I felt very angry and depressed. I didn't go out of my house at all. I couldn't make myself get out of bed except to use the rest room. During all my waking hours I relived every moment of humiliation Bo created for me. My mind was so full of *should of's and could of's.*

Jeff is very supportive. He treats me like his queen even though I felt and looked like a rag-a-muffin. We sat down and talked out our financial situation and he wrote out four or five budgets. Each one came out in the red. We weren't quite certain how we were going to financially make ends meet. We prayed together and tried not to take our frustrations out on each other. Sometimes it worked and sometimes it didn't.

I applied for unemployment benefits. Thank God the Court of Claims didn't fight that. Standing in the unemployment line reminded me of the food stamp line. It felt so unfair. I wasn't suppose to be doing this. I'm the victim. And all I could think of was Bo in his newly appointed position with the governor, sitting in his high-back leather chair behind a mahogony stained desk with a glass top and name plate that says, Bo Gilyard, Director. It looks like he's sailing pretty high. I knew that he had no care or concern about the pain and financial anguish he had just caused me and my family. He was too busy breaking in his new throne and probably establishing his authority as *Head Nigger In Charge.* I knew that Mike and Jack were unbothered too. It did not effect them at all. I was angry that I didn't get to say good-bye to my co-workers and let them know what really happened. I felt that it was a shame that no one would ever know the truth. I felt so many different things and it had me so tense and tight and with the worst case of diarrhea I've had in a long time. My appetite, needless to say was buried and forgotten. I'm already slim, now I look like skin and bones.

Journal Entry XXIX

I woke up with an urgent thought on my mind. "I must get some help". This pain I was feeling was giving me bad dreams at night. Although I felt like shit warmed over, I had a strong will to survive. But I didn't quite know how to help myself. I knew I had to find somebody to show me the way. But who?

I looked in the telephone book and found an organization called, Committee Against Sexual Harassment, (C.A.S.H.). I called and left a message. I know I must have sounded pretty desperate. I was. The lady who called me back had so much concern in her voice. Her name was Judi Moseley. She listened very compassionately to my story and without judgement. She told me about C.A.S.H. and invited me out to their next meeting. I shared with her the physical symptoms I was suffering from and the guilt I was feeling. Judi suggested that I may want to consider getting therapy to help me handle my stress. I told her that I did not want to talk my pain over with a male doctor. She gave me the names of three female professionals she recommended. Said that they could be very helpful. I called, and one was on vacation for two weeks, the other two did not take the insurance coverage I had. Since I didn't have a job, I couldn't afford their fees. I kept looking and asking around to no avail. I asked Judi about lawyers too. I told her that I had plans to file a charge with the Civil Rights Commission. I was making a conscious decision to stand on what was, "Good, just, and righteous". I felt that I was well versed enough on how to write a charge. Jeff could help. He's my dependable support.

I called Commission and was given an appointment to file a charge of sexual harassment with the Commission. In the mean time, I was still looking for a therapist to help me with my depression. Seems like Bo brought to surface some unresolved issues I had buried regarding my former abusive marriage to Arthur. I was hurting all over again on the inside just like I use to back then. This time I wanted to fix it and not bury it. This time I'll get help to start my long overdue healing process.

Finally, after nearly a two month wait, my appointment with the Commission arrived...

PART II

THE
CHARGE

Sexual
Harassment
Filing

CHARGE OF DISCRIMINATION

(Individual's real names are omitted)

Issue I:

~ I am a Black female who was employed a field coordinator for the Court of Claims of Ohio, Victims of Crime Program from approximately July 29, 1990 through January 31, 1991, at which time I was terminated.

~ The Director of the Victims of Crime Program was Mr. "A" and he hired me. Mr. "A" repeatedly made lewd remarks about me, touched me, and commented about my physical features.

~ On or about January 25, 1991, Mr. "A" was appointed as Director of the Governor's Office of Criminal Justice Services. He called the Clerk of Court of Claims, Mr. "B", and told him to fire me. I asked Mr. "B" why I was being fired and Mr. "B" told me Mr. "A", your supervisor, recommended that you be terminated. I was not disciplined, nor aware of any unsatisfactory job performance and not given a mid or final performance evaluation.

Issue II:

~ I believe I have been unlawfully discriminated against due to Mr. "A"'s consideration of my sex, female, race, Black and sexual harassment, insomuch as I, as well as other females, were sexually harassed by Mr. "A", Black male.

Issue III:

~ On or about November 15, 1990, Mr. "A" instructed me to go to Cleveland, Ohio to a conference with him. He asked me out to dinner during the night of our arrival. He told me during dinner that he has a phobia regarding driving over bridges. The doctor gave him medication that made him "impotent' and he had not had a "hard-on" in a long time. He stopped taking the medication so that he could get a "hard on" and now he is back to normal. After dinner, we went back to the hotel. He walked me to my room and talked for about 15-20 minutes in front of my room door. He kept starring at me, looking at me up and down. I finally left and I called my husband and told him I felt uncomfortable around Mr. "A". He invited me to breakfast the next morning and starting telling me sexual jokes which included the following:

a. There was a guy named "Long Dick Willie". His dick was 10 feet long and his dick scared women away. He tried women on the east and west coast and women would always run from his big dick. One day out of frustration, "Long Dick Willie" cried and complained to his best friend. His friend arranged for him to meet a woman who could take every inch of his dick. He met the woman and they began to "fuck". Willie was afraid she would not be able to handle his long dick so he eased it to her slowly. Much to his surprise, she kept saying more, more, more and Long Dicked Willie had finally met the perfect pussy and he asked her how does it feel she responded (at this point, Mr. "A" quickly stuck his tongue in and out to indicate that Long Dick Willie's penis had come up through her throat and was moving in and out of her mouth) then he, Mr. "A", started laughing and starting telling another joke:

b. This fellow suspected that his wife was cheating on him so he hired a hit man to follow her and catch her in the act. The hit man was instructed to shoot his wife in the middle of the head and to shoot his wife's lover in the balls. The hit man said, "fine, but I charge $1,000 for each bullet I have to use." They agreed upon $2,000. The husband and the hit man followed the wife and her lover to a hotel and they watched them enter the room together. They were so anxious to start "fucking" that they forgot to close the window blinds so the hit man could see them very well through the telescope on his rifle. The hit man began to describe to the husband what they were doing. He said they were kissing and feeling all over one another and how they fell onto the bed. The husband shouted out, "What are you waiting for, shoot them!" The hit man said, just be patient, if you just wait a minute, she's going down one him, I can get you two for the price of one bullet."

c. There was a nerd who could never get a date to go to bed with him because every time he would take off his clothes the women would laugh at him because his dick was so tiny. On New Years Eve he was all by himself in a lonely hotel room. He thought about getting laid and began to make a wish. His wish was so sincere that a genie appeared and said that he would grant the nerd one free wish. Since the nerd never had sex before, that was all he could think of as being the one thing he really, really wanted. And he thought that if he had a penis like a "nigger", women would have sex with him. So he said, "I wish I was 'hung like a nigger'. The genie said, "Your wish is my command," and disappeared. The nerd was quite anxious for his change to come and he waited and waited and kept looking at his dick but he saw no change. Finally, he heard a knock at the door, he saw three large men with white hoods on their head holding a noose and they said, "Are you the one who wanted to be hung like a nigger?"

~ I was surprised as Mr. "A" continuously talked to me about sex. When we returned to Columbus, Ohio, I told my husband that Mr. "A" was always talking about sex and I feel uncomfortable around him. My husband asked me if I wanted him to have a word with him about it and I said no because Mr. "A"'s ego is real sensitive and he might take it out on me some more. So he suggested that I tell Mr. "A" how his behavior offended me and asked him to stop because his actions could be perceived as sexual harassment.

I did and I also told him that his screaming and cursing at me made me feel uncomfortable. His jaws began to twitch and could see that what I said made him very angry. He started banging down on his desk and started pointing his finger and talking to me very rudely. He said "Goddamit, Patricia, this is my court and I run things around here, not the Clerk, not the Supreme Court Justice or the Supreme Court Judges. This is my Court and if you do not get that through your thick head, then you need to find something else to do. I pay your salary. Before I hired you, you weren't nothing. If you would act right, I had big plans for you. Do you understand English!" I was hurt and shaken and was only able to respond, "I'm listening." He insisted on a different response and I finally said, "Yes Sir, Yes Boss." Then he calmly said, "Now get out and get back to work."

Issue IV

~ After the trip from Cleveland, Mr. "A" indicated that I would never go out of town with him, because I should be home taking care of my husband. He indicated that I should have given into his desires. He told me I had a pretty ass on several occasions. He also told my co-worker, Mr. "C" and the staff attorney, now Director of the Victims of Crime Program, Mr. "D", that I had the prettiest ass in the Court.

~ He told me that he hated his mother and that I reminded him of his first wife who was a crazy bitch.

~ During the ministerial breakfast in Cleveland, Ohio, in October, 1990, I took a picture with Supreme Court Chief Justice and Mr. "B", Clerk of the Court of Claims. The pictures were developed for the Court of Claims. He tore up, burned and threw away the picture with me, Chief Justice and the Clerk.

~ During the ministerial breakfast, Mr. "A" gave a speech and belittled women during his speech regarding domestic violence. Ms. "G", then candidate for Judge, brought the afore to his attention during the question and answer session because she and other females in the audience were offended. When we returned back to the office, he told me and other co-workers that he hates that black ugly bitch and if he had a gun, he would shoot her.

Issue V.

Mr. "A" would began to yell, scream and curse at me on such a regular basis that I was very stressed and would cry because of the way he made me feel. It had gotten so bad that I began to confide in one of my co-workers, Mr. "C" and one day we had lunch and talked about Mr. "A"'s rude behavior towards. Mr. "C" asked me if I had promised Mr. "A" sex because he talked about my "ass" all the time and he's always cutting me down for no apparent reason. Mr. "C" said I must not be giving him any play and that's why I was having problems.

Issue VI

On approximately November 7, around 3:00p.m., I went to Mr. "A"'s office to give him the status of a project and the door was closed. As I approached the door, I could hear noises and laughter. Ms. "L", his secretary said that maybe I should knock because Mr. "A" was sitting in front of the door. I knocked and peeked in and saw Mr. "A", Mr. "R", (staff attorney) and Mr. "C" sitting around the video/television player and they had surprised looks on their face. I stated that I came up to give him an update but that I would come back later.

I saw Mr. "C" later and he stated that Mr. "A" was sitting in front of the door to block any surprise entrances. Much to Mr. "C"'s surprise, Mr. "A", Director, was in his office viewing X-rated movies with Mr. "R". Mr. "C" said the film showed a lot of "ass action". He felt uncomfortable but knew Mr. "A" Director, did not want him to leave.

Issue VII

~ When I or Ms. "L", his secretary would eat a banana or oblong donut, Mr. "A",Director would tell us that we look good with the item in our mouths.

~ Director "A" also asked me during a staff meeting what Church I attended. I said Mt. Hermon, and he replied, "Oh, you go where that _____ preacher goes, Dr. "W"."

Issue VIII

He would touches me and tries to hug me - I would try to avoid and resist contact with him.

Issue IX

~ He prohibited me from talking with the Clerk of the Court of Claims, Mr. "B". Mr. "A" told me that I had better not answer any questions Mr. "B" may ask me concerning any projects that Mr. "A" assigned. Mr. "A" told me to play or put Mr. "B" off because he is a real "fuck-up". He often referred to the Clerk as "Spuds" or "butt head" during our morning staff meetings. When the Clerk would come into the morning meetings, Mr. "A" would say something disrespectful and negative about Mr. "B" after he left and would roll his eyes up in his head in disgust.

Issue X

~ During one of our morning staff meetings, Mr. "A" stated that the larger the boobs, the dumber the woman so that means that Carson, Ms. "L", and Ms. "P" should be real smart. We were the only women present.

Issue XI

Mr. "A" received an appointment to another Directorship. He called the new Director and the Clerk of the Court of Claims and told them to terminate me.

Surprisingly, the Civil Rights Commission accepted my written charge without making many changes. They said my case would be assigned and that I would be notified regarding its progress.

PART III

OBTAINING
GOOD
LEGAL
HELP

Interrogatories

THINGS TO CONSIDER

      After drafting my own charges and filing a sexual harassment charge with the Civil Rights Commission and the Equal Employment

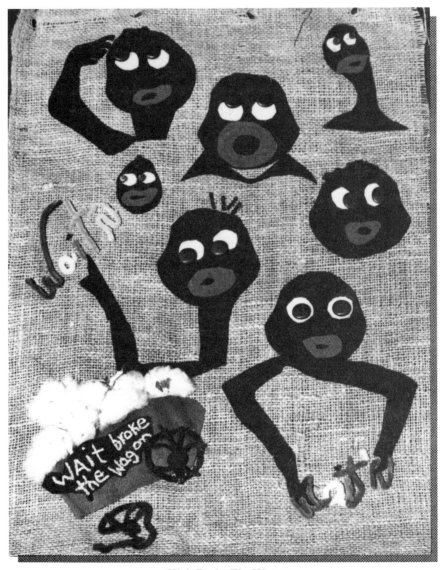

Wait Broke The Wagon

Opportunity Commission, I waited and waited and waited for justice. I called several times and spoke with my case worker. He told me that the charged party did not have a time frame in which to respond to my charge of sexual harassment. Further, he said that I had to wait until they responded no matter how long it took. I knew that was not true, but his answer told me two things. 1) That as an employee of the Ohio Civil Rights Commission, he was not going to be very helpful in getting me justice and 2) That I had better start looking for an attorney. In order to get my case turned over to private counsel, I had to obtain a "Right to Sue Letter" from the Ohio Civil Rights Commission. I was told that this letter was like a written permission slip to bring legal action against the government. Something to do with sovereign immunity. After numerous sincere attempts to obtain my "Right To Sue Letter", I finally succeeded and officially hired an attorney. I was determined not to wait any longer! Grandma Leon use to say, "Wait? Wait for what? Wait broke the wagon! Face your fears now or they'll be lookin' at you later!"

There are several things to consider if you are interested in filing your own law suit against your harasser. Know that you will be playing hard ball. Be certain that it is your decision to go forward and not someone else. You will be the primary person responsible for the outcome.

A civil law suit can take years. Many people who start off in support of your efforts will soon be involved in their own day to day survival. So you must be willing to go at it alone if necessary.

Please take time to read through the suggestions I offer and take my hard learned lessons to heart.

...I waited and waited on the Commission to help me get my job back. The individual who was assigned my case appeared to have no intention of going up against the Supreme Court on my behalf. After a more than reasonable wait for a response from the Court, I obtained a Right to Sue Letter and officially hired an attorney. The attorney agreed upon a retainer's fee of $500. Jeff and I scraped that amount up from somewhere and hired him.

By this time, I was traveling back and forth to Dayton on the weekends for therapy sessions with Dr. Bond. She was willing to provide counseling sessions for me until such time as I was able to pay. Her therapy helped me tremendously. She provided me with tools that helped me help myself. I had so much coming at me at once, on top of being broke with no money, I was also broken on the inside.

Today, my attorney tells me that the Attorney General is summoning me to appear in a deposition hearing. I was not prepared for what was about to happen to me. I was hoping that the two highest law officials in the State of Ohio, the Supreme Court and the Attorney General, would surely not drag their feet on such a blatant act of sexual harassment as this. But I was fooled. And if a victim can ever be revictimized, it can happen at a deposition. The interrogating sessions at a deposition can be very devastating. I was required to answer personal questions, even with regards to my previous marriage.

No one told me that depositions were another form of harassment. And what is even more frightening, I was told by my attorney that this type of harassment was legal. There are no laws in place that specifically address and protect a victim against the type of questioning, the amount of questioning, or the badgering that can arise during deposition sessions. The mannerisms that are displayed during depositions are directly in line with the individuals that are conducting the interrogation and their motives.

It was quite obvious that the Attorney General's office and the Court of Claims were not interested in justice. A party who is not interested in the truth and making the victim legally whole can damage the victim even more. And that's what was happening with me. Plus I could not adequately defend my right to due process because I could not afford it. I was being punished for speaking out against the breaking of the law that these same law official were voted into office to uphold. They were not enforcing their own laws.

I hadn't felt so helpless in a long, long time. I felt like Daniel must have felt when he was thrown into a den of vicious, hungry lions. He had done no wrong. He was just outspoken with the truth of his faith and belief. He refused to be silenced. So the powers that be sentenced him to a hideous death. He was sentenced to be ripped and torn apart by hungry lions in a den where thousands before him had been unjustly murdered. Biblical history tells us, that as the public watched in anticipation of the victim's demise, some would cheer in ignorance, not knowing that they too were victims. Others would look on in fear, knowing that a grave injustice was being carried out. Yet both were too afraid to come to the defense of the unjustly condemned; too conditioned to think that their voice of rebellion could make a difference. Their faith had been shaken too many times before and perhaps they too had suffered the torturous addicts of their slave masters, for they were in mental bondage.

But Daniel, like myself had been called unto a higher calling. In our flesh we were weakened by the mere thought of torment, but within our spirits, we knew that God would never forsake us. Like Daniel, I too sang the Lord's praises, and like Daniel, I had psalms of deliverance on my tongue.

The den of lions I was summoned to go before today was the Attorney General. They deposed me over and over again to question my claim that Bo had sexually harassed me and that I was terminated based on sex discrimination.

My sister Toni attended a deposition hearing with me. It did me good to know that she was in the room. Her presence gave me strength. Fifteen minutes into the questioning, one of the Assistant Attorney General made a formal request for Toni to be removed from the proceedings. They said that since I had previously discussed with her my sexual harassment claim against Bo Gilyard, she may be called upon to be a witness. Therefore, she could not remain in the proceedings. She was all I had that day and without her I did not feel that I could handle another eight hours of badgering.

I cried and they took a recess. In the hallway, Toni just hugged me and tried to get me to clear my mind about the whole situation. She said, "They are just trying to wear you down and discourage you, but you must remain strong. God and truth is on your side. You are not the criminal here. Hold your head up and know that this battle is already won!"

She didn't leave the building, she sat in a room across from the hearing and waited. When I finished with the deposition session, she handed me a very uplifting message she had written while waiting. She said, "When you get home, put this day behind you. Run yourself a nice, warm Calgon bubble bath and put on some nice, soft music and just soak. After that, find yourself a quiet spot and read this letter I wrote. I think you just need to be reminded of how special you are."

When I got home, I followed her directions to the "T". Her letter was so inspiring...

Dear Patricia:

God never said what he needs for his followers to do would be easy. After all, the Bible is full of the trials and tribulations of the righteous that chose to stand against darkness. There appears to be much darkness for you now. It will be. Can't you see the devil is running scared. Remember, the Creator has the power over it all!

The adversary is a liar and a picture painter. He has painted his followers (victims) a portrait of deception. Be proud you have been chosen to see it for what it really is. Many cannot.

There's no need to cry for yourself. It is a gift from God to be able to see. If you must weep, weep for those who cannot see. You've received a victory! It's already been won on the spiritual plane. The rest is just the conclusion of a long story already told.

But wait! There's more. There always will be; for the devil is busy. You've been assigned your duty because you have chosen the light. There is no time to rest. Your resting days are over. Stop letting the devil fool you that your peace of mind and rest comes from starving yourself and lying in your bed of depression. That's his picture for you. That is not the image God created for you. There is joy in the morning because God woke you up and there is joy at night because he brought you through the day.

Stop feeling sorry for yourself. So what if the adversary chose to speak out against you. Would you rather them speak for you? If they did, you would need to take a closer look at yourself in the mirror and question who you really serve.

Welcome the challenges and welcome being a child who chose to serve her Creator, the almighty of not some, but of all living things.

Love, your sister Toni

I carried Toni's letter with me as a reminder of my greatness. I was truly forced to walk by faith and not my sight. And every time

I wavered out of my faith mode, I was emerged in total fear because I appeared to be out numbered, out spent; out equipped, out smarted, out maneuvered, out ranked, and out weighed. As a result, I sometimes would feel out-of-balance, outraged, out stretched, and out worn. Many days I felt like an outcast. All because, I was outspoken.

When I concentrated on my circumstances too long I became outraged because my tax dollars, my husband's tax dollars, my mother and father's tax dollars, my grandparents tax dollars, my children's tax dollars; (five generation of tax payers dollars), and all the tax payers in the state of Ohio were paying for Bo's defense. It would have cost the state less if they accepted the legal responsibility of upholding the laws they were elected or appointed to enforce, and give me my job back.

Be aware that...

Even though you are the victim, you may end up as the defendant. You may be forced to defend your character, your past actions in past relationships, your professional ethics, and all of your feelings, thoughts, words, actions and reaction in response to your harasser's alleged behavior towards you. Stay strong.

During my depositions, I was subjected to days of one hour after another of interrogation. You may have to give written reply to pre-deposition questions, called interrogatories.

[Interrogatories such as:]

Interrogatory Number 1:

Please identify each item of damage and the amount of each such item that you allege was caused by defendant's conduct. Such identification should include, but not be limited to the items mentioned in each claim of your complaint and in the prayer for relief, including the economic loss, present and future, emotional injury, and any punitive damages you are now claiming or may claim in the future.

Interrogatory Number 2:

Identify each person who, to your knowledge, information or belief, has any knowledge of any of the facts or circumstances relating to your responses to the preceding interrogatory, or the facts upon which you base your response, and, for each person so identified, set forth all such knowledge you know, believe or are informed that person possesses.

Interrogatory Number 3:

With respect to your claims in Paragraphs 18 and 25 of the Complaint that you suffered grave emotional distress, humiliation and embarrassment, state the name, address and telephone number of any doctor, psychiatrist, psychologist or other person who has examined, treated, counseled, or consulted with you for such injury or distress, the dates of such treatment, the costs of such treatment, and a description of the manifestation and diagnoses relative to such emotional injury.

104

Interrogatory Number 4:

Do you contend that you have suffered any damages other than those set forth in response to Interrogatory Number 17? If your answer is anything other than an unqualified "no," set forth each and every item, a description of each item and the amount of such additional damage which you contend you have suffered.

Interrogatory Number 5:

Identify each person who, to your knowledge, information or belief, has any knowledge of any of the facts or circumstances relating to your response to the preceding interrogatory, or the facts upon which you base your response, and, for each so identified, set forth all such knowledge you know, believe or are informed that person possesses.

Interrogatory Number 6:

Describe each action which you have taken or which you plan to take, if any, to mitigate any of the damages suffered by you due to your termination by Victims of Crime?

Interrogatory Number 7:

Describe all efforts you have taken to find employment subsequent to your termination by Victims of Crime. This description should include, but not be limited to, the following: the names, addresses and telephone numbers of the prospective employers you have contacted; the date(s) you sought employment from each prospective employer; the position whether you received an offer of employment from such employer and, if not, the reason for your rejection if it was expressed to you.

Interrogatory Number 8:

For each employer for whom you have worked subsequent to your termination by Victims of Crime, please state the following; the name, address and telephone number of the employer, the title or position you held; the compensation you received (per pay period and in total); a description of all fringe benefits offered by or received from such employer, including but not limited to, medical insurance, life insurance, pension or retirement benefits or profit sharing; the reason, if any you left such employment; and, the date you began and/or ended employment with such employer.

Interrogatory Number 9:

Describe each fact or belief, conversation or other oral or written communication upon which you base your contention that you were discriminated against in whole or in part because of your race.

Interrogatory Number 10:

Identify each person that you know or believe to have information relating to your performance or termination as an employee of Victims of Crime and state all the knowledge or information you know or believe that person possesses relating to those subjects which you believe supports or evidences the allegations in the Complaints or the facts upon which you base such allegations.

Interrogatory Number 11:

List and describe with specificity each and every fact or belief, circumstance, conversation or other oral or written communicate upon which you base your belief in Paragraph of the Complaint that you were wrongfully discharged "due to plaintiff's refusal to submit to supervisor's sexual demands."

Interrogatory Number 12:

With respect to Paragraph 18 of your Complaint, please set forth the factual basis for your allegation that "(t)he unconsented physical control, sexual demands, abusive language, and wrongful discharge by Gilyard was willful, wanton, malicious and outrageous."

Interrogatory Number 13:

Describe each fact or belief upon which you base your contention that "Gilyard had previously engaged in sexually harassing conduct with other female employees of the Ohio Court of Claims" as alleged in Paragraph 14 of your Complaint.

...these were just some of the questions I had to answer. The Actual deposition went on for several days spread out over weeks. Sometimes up to eight hours per day.

I've included these interrogatories (questions) for your deep consideration to any valid claims you may have in a civil filing. Please be mentally and physically prepared to withstand the vigorous line of questioning that is going to be put to you. Along with that may come false and misleading statements that will be made against you. Many times there will be no way for you to disprove them. It is during those times that you will feel victimized all over again. But be strong, seek help and stay prayerful. If at anytime you feel it is costing you your health, please reconsider other strategies. Nothing is worth your health, your life. Women have committed suicide behind this type of pressure and many have experienced failed health. Make wise decisions. Don't be surprised when people from your own race call you a traitor for speaking out against one of your own. When that happened to me, I calmly asked, "Where were you were when I was getting abused, or why didn't you speak up for me when I needed you the most? And if I don't speak out against injustice, who will? You should ask yourself the same question. That's exactly how evil continues to exists -- enough good people do absolutely nothing!"

Even though I could not monetarily afford the due process the law said I had a right to and in the midst of what appeared to be lack, God's infinite supply of my needs never ceased; nor did God's presence forsake me. I remember one particular time God really reminded me of my blessed position. As a believer, I am one of the protected.

I had just finished listening to my attorney tell me that his firm did not purchase transcripts from deposition. He said that I would have to order and pay for any transcripts used in my case preparation. I told him that I had no job! I can't even barely afford to buy gas to put in the car to get to the deposition let alone purchase the transcripts of my depositions at $2 or $3 per page. Then I asked him how on earth he could prepare for my trial without important facts that come out of the depositions? He said that he took notes and would do fine without them. That just didn't seem like enough to me. Especially when I was up against the highest judicial system in the State of Ohio, the Court of Claims, which is administered by the Supreme Court of Ohio. Good, solid, preparation was essential.

I had no one to turn to but God, and I lay across my bed and cried and then cleared my mind and talked to God straight from the heart and told God what was going on and how helpless I felt. Then I just lay there waiting for my answer.

The telephone rang. I didn't want to be disturbed, so I just let it ring. But the phone would not stop ringing so I picked it up. On the other end of the line was a voice that sounded soft, concerned, and sincere. She said her name was Cheryl and she asked to speak with Patricia Wingard Carson. I said that I was Patricia, and then she said that she did not quite understand why she was doing this, but that she believed that a person in my position should be able to afford their defense and that she was being spiritually obedient. She asked for my address because, she said, that she wanted to send me, by certified mail, transcripts of the two deposition hearings she recorded regarding my case, free of charge.

I was speechless and kept telling her over and over thank you, thank you, thank you. She had no idea how much her spiritual obedience has blessed me and reminded me that I am not alone, that God is the determining factor in this matter.

So no, I could not afford to hire an attorney that had

resources to purchase what was needed in preparation of my trial nor did he have an investigative staff that could collect the facts and evidence to substantiate my claim. Jeff and I had to do much of my investigative work. Although I have an extensive background in investigations, under the many other stresses I was experiencing, it was very difficult for me to concentrate my efforts on my case. There were many, many other demands I had to fulfill each day and it was becoming next to impossible to be in three places at one time. We only had one automobile and my husband often needed it to get to work. If I were able to keep the car for the day, I had very little or no money for gas. The bottom line, is this, I was being punished for something I did not do. My job was taken away from me for something I did not do. The entire income of my household was cut in half without notice for something I did not do. And now I am required to get further in debt to defend myself, for something I did not do! But through it all, I learned to trust in God's word even more. Every now and then, God would remind me that this was not my battle and that victory had already been won. All I needed to do was to hold out and keep walking by faith, not by sight.

God and I not only had to not only stay ever ready to respond to the Attorney General's request, but I had to subject myself to the hard times that come with unemployment, i.e. standing in the unemployment lines, week after week; looking for another job and having to explain what happen with my last employment; financial stress; and the physical illness that comes along with stress. But the pain of not being believed was the deepest.

Finally, I realized that it was not an issue of belief. But one of accountability. Eventually, the facts became clear enough to substantiate my claim. But the justice system still did not choose accept their legal responsibility.

But God will not be mocked!

Brief outline of Bo's demise:

April 19, 1991 - I filed a sexual harassment charge, against Gilyard with the Ohio Civil Rights Commission. A letter had previously been remitted to top law officials, including the Supreme Court Chief Justice outlining Gilyard's conduct. There appeared to be no response. Eventually I filed private charges.

July 19, 1991 - Gilyard was charged with the allegation of *theft in office* and he was placed on administrative leave, (Allegation: non-state business trips with hotels stay(s) for the purpose of having sex).

July 22, 1991 - Gilyard's alleged active participation in the mistreatment (beating) of six youths during his employment as a Youth Leader was revealed. It was said that Gilyard had failed to provide the extent of his involvement during his background check regarding his appointment to the governor's cabinet. A determination was made to terminate Gilyard from his $63,500-a-year position.

In an effort to save his job, Gilyard made allegations that he had been fired for providing information on the alleged ethical misconduct of high state officials. His allegations placed top official under the scope. Gilyard fought with everything he had to no avail. He searched for vindication high and low. But he forgot a few crucial factors:

~ The experience he was going through was not controlled by man. God was at work now. He was reaping what he had sown. The immutable laws of the universe were in motion. And as my pastor, Dr. Washington says, "When God opens a door, it can not be shut by no man. And when God shuts a door it can not be opened by no man." Bo's evil seeds of pain were ripe for harvest.

~ The Inspector General's report found Gilyard's actions and personality to be very much like my testament.

~ As a result of this high profile case, Bo's picture, name, and many other shocking details made news headlines throughout the entire State of Ohio for several months to come. He found himself to be quite friendless. In one article, Bo was quoted as making reference to how he's relies on God and how his faith has grown.

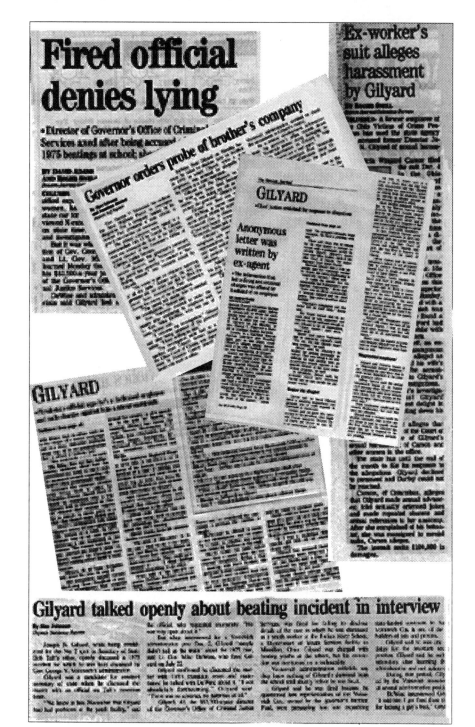

Reprinted with the permission of the Columbus (Ohio) Dispatch and the Akron Beacon Journal

Unfortunately, I was still going through the results of my law suit. But once they found my sexual harassment charge against Bo to have merit, they resorted to attacking my professional character and continued to victimize me. I guess, the instant I began to complained, I became *retroactively incompetent.*

Even Supreme Court Chief Justice Douglas J. Morton, who I was told appointed Gilyard to his position in the Court of Claims wrote off my complaint as insignificant.

In a reply letter addressed to the Inspector General regarding the Inspector General's inquiry into Gilyard being charged with the sexual harassment of a female employee (me) of the Court of Claims, Chief Justice Morton stated, *"I am convinced after talking with Mr. Gilyard, as I was certain before discussing the matter with him, that he is not engaged in any inappropriate conduct as alleged..."*

I was written off as a disgruntled employee with inadequate performance. Chief Justice Morton's written position was very disheartening.

Then another surprise was thrown my way. [And I suggest you stay prepared for surprises. Good ones and bad ones]. During my deposition I was asked to identify a letter that was offered as State Exhibit. This letter was written on the Court of Claims of Ohio letterhead and signed by then Court appointed director, Bo Gilyard.

When I began to read this letter and I was floored! This letter stated that I had been terminated not because I had been sexually

115

harassed and had refused the advances of my harasser, but because I was *actively violent, incompetent, and non-cooperative.* I was informed at my deposition that the Public Information Officer of the Court of Claims, Lillian Brewster, volunteered to write this letter for Bo. Bo was more than happy to sign-off on it. All lies! I found myself defending my professional character against lies. I had to fight to keep this false document from being permanently placed in my personnel file. I would never be able to explain that behavior to any future prospective employer who made inquiry into my employment history.

This letter was marked as State Exhibit and entered into evidence. It didn't matter that it was a lie. Not only was I not violent, I never even raised my voice in the Court or had words with anyone but Bo. And those words were mild. Too mild! If you asked anyone who knows me to describe my character, the words *violent, incompetent, and non-cooperative* would never be thought of. Those three words described the total opposite of my demeanor.

...more

It's very essential that you establish a strong support base. This could be family, friends, church affiliates, organizations who address women's issues, or other survivors. *The Committee Against Sexual Harassment*, which was founded by Judi Moseley, and four other women in Columbus, Ohio, was very helpful to me.

It is important that you do not be afraid or ashamed to tell your story and seek help. Even though I thought I was handling my stress well, I wasn't. All I was doing was internalizing it and producing serious physical and psychological challenges for myself. I ended up on medication for stress induced vertigo and in therapy. When I finally realized I was falling apart, I searched high and low for counseling/therapy. Even in my fragmented state of mind, I was determined to find a female therapist. At the time, I felt men could not understand my pain. I ended up driving back and forth to Dayton, Ohio to have therapy sessions with Dr. Giovonni Bond. She was a life saver in more ways than one.

When hiring legal help:

Many of the lawyers I talked to wanted a substantial retainer's fee, some as high as $10,000. Others didn't want to take on my case at all because the Court that harassed me was administered by the Ohio Supreme Court. The Supreme Court plays a very important role in determining who practices law in the State of Ohio and who does not. So rocking the boat was too risky for some lawyers.

Ideally, I wanted to be represented by an Afrikan American attorney. Someone who would be brave, bold, and expert enough to get me justice. It became very frustrating - but I didn't give up. An associate recommended an Afrikan American attorney that was new to the city. I was so worn-out that I didn't shop around for legal representation as well as I should have.

I called and made an appointment to discuss my case with this attorney. He said that he had successfully litigated sexual harassment cases and convinced me that he could handle my case all the way to the end. We agreed upon a retainer fee of $500 and one-third of any and all monies received from the law suit.

Here's what I learned from my experience:

~When looking for good solid representation, disregard race and gender.

~Before hiring your attorney, make certain the person you are considering is *really* an expert in sexual harassment litigation. Ask for proof of past case history and look at their litigation success rate. That's the bottom line. That's where the rubber meets the road!

~Ideally, you want an attorney who has vast resources that are immediately available to him or her. For example, an investigative staff to assist with the fact-gathering process; experienced researchers of case law; an operating budget so that potential critical witnesses can be deposed and their transcripts can be purchased so that your attorney can utilize this important information to help in the preparation of your case, etc..

~Stay away from attorneys whose case load is so heavy that they cannot provide you adequate representation. It does not matter how great their skills are. If they do not have time to apply their skills to your case, it does you no good!

~Make certain you obtain an attorney who listens to you. You know your experience better then anyone. Your attorney should be able to listen to your story and determine the proper legalese to use in preparing your case.

~Find out if your attorney is obligated in any way to the parties you are bringing charges against. This sometimes includes, friendships, associations, business affiliations, etc.. It can cause clouded thinking and may seriously effect their judgement of the real issue(s) at hand.

~Your attorney should be willing to represent you all the way and not pressure you into settlement before you are ready. There are others principles involved other than money. Your case could be the case to change laws and help to put a stop to sexual harassment, or at least make it more costly to the perpetrators.

~Make certain you have an attorney who is timely in responding not only to you but to legal inquiries concerning your case. Timely filing of legal documents could be critical.

~If your harasser terminated you and you want your job back, or if your harasser was physically abusive to you, or whatever you particular case may be, make certain that your attorney is willing and able to present your case, your position, and protect your constitutional rights.

~Ask your attorney up front exactly what his or her fees are, and what their fees cover. Surprise cost factors can cause you to lose your case if you are not financially able to cover the cost of due process. Once the terms are outlined, sign an agreement with your attorney and keep a copy for your files.

~Keep copies of everything regarding your case and maintain your own organized files. Some attorneys may make it difficult for you to obtain your case files from them after your case has ended and they have gotten paid.

~The most important aspect in picking legal counsel is to follow your intuition and know that your attorney believes in your case. Make certain that he or she has a "zealous approach" in representing you as required within their oath. Passion for principle goes a long ways. Know that if you are standing on truth, God is on your side and your battle is already won! But don't forget to work your case as if everything depends upon you and pray as if everything depends upon God.... it does.

My life now...

The State of Ohio and I did reach a monetary settlement agreement regarding my sexual harassment law suit. I didn't get my job back though and it took me two whole years to find another job. But I prevailed in so many other ways.

Although my new job as an investigator in the health field,

paid much less than when I was a field coordinator with the Ohio Victims of Crime Compensation Program, I am grateful to be out of the unemployment line. I'm not certain that I'll never feel comfortable or secure within any job though. Whether we want to admit it or not, often our career advancements are influenced by the personality traits of others and how we choose to interact. So I've learned to depend upon my Creator to place me where I should be. It does feel quite good, however, to work in an environment where I am not judged by my waist-line or breast size.

Some people ask me if I had it to do all over again would I still file a law suit and what would I do different if I did.

The answer is, "Yes." There are a few things I would do differently: I would make my law suit more public; I would be more critical in my research for an attorney; I would insist that my attorney file my case in federal court instead of in the same court, the Court of Claims, where I was victimized; I would stay in closer contact with all my family members and friends instead of shutting myself off from them; and I would definitely be kinder and more gentle with myself.

God has continued be a blessing in my life. My family and I just recently moved into our first new home. Jeff and I have worked hard to get our finances back in order. We're still working on them. We have learned to be more patient with each other and we try not to sweat the small stuff. A lot of sacrifices were made during my law suit, but all in all, we developed a deeper appreciation for one another and our faith in God certainly did grow. I'm a stronger and wiser person because of this experience.

All three of our sons, Dorian, Derrick and Christopher, have entered adulthood and are either employed or in college. We hope our lives will serve as an example to them and to those who witnessed the triumph of our challenge. This entire experience has served to bring us closer together.

We are grateful to family, friends, and everyone who was instrumental in supporting us.

I continue to conduct workshops and seminars on various topics; one being sexual harassment issues, now that I've established quite a bit of expertise.

I have testified before the Ohio Senate in support of Senator Jeffrey Johnson's Bill against sexual harassment and I'm an on-going volunteer with the Committee Against Sexual Harassment. I don't run around preaching *the sexual harassment gospel as told by Patricia Wingard Carson*, but I do continue to stand up for what the Creator places on my heart as being -- good, just, and righteous.

~~~~~~~[]~~~~~~~

Last I heard, Bo was trying to make a living selling used cars.

~~~~~~~[]~~~~~~~

PART IV

OTHER
HELPFUL
INFORMATION

The Committee Against Sexual Harassment was very informative. Some of the important information they provided for me is outlined on the following pages. It is provided with the written permission of the Committee Against Sexual Harassment.

SEXUAL HARASSMENT DEFINITION:

Legal Definition: Based on TITLE VII of the 1964 Civil Rights Act; Taken from the Equal Employment Opportunity Commission (EEOC) Guidelines issued in November, 1980.

UNWELCOME SEXUAL ADVANCES, REQUESTS FOR SEXUAL FAVORS, AND OTHER VERBAL OR PHYSICAL CONDUCT OF A SEXUAL NATURE CONSTITUTE SEXUAL HARASSMENT WHEN:

1) SUBMISSION TO SUCH CONDUCT IS MADE EITHER EXPLICITLY OR IMPLICITLY A TERM OR CONDITION OF AN INDIVIDUAL'S;

2) SUBMISSION TO OR REJECTION OF SUCH CONDUCT BY AN INDIVIDUAL IS USED AS THE BASIS FOR EMPLOYMENT DECISIONS AFFECTING SUCH INDIVIDUALS; OR

3) SUCH CONDUCT HAS THE PURPOSE OR EFFECT OF UNREASONABLY INTERFERING WITH AN INDIVIDUAL'S WORK PERFORMANCE OR CREATING AN INTIMIDATING, HOSTILE, OR OFFENSIVE WORKING ENVIRONMENT.

THE EEOC:

1. Considers each case individually.

2. Generally holds the employer responsible for the acts of employees. The employer may also be held

responsible for the acts of non-employees such as individuals making deliveries or performing repair work.

3.   Will look for signs of preventive measures and signs of other discrimination.

4.   Can seek back pay, reinstatement, promotion, good letters of recommendation, no reprisals, or other denied benefits.

The Ohio Civil Rights Commission (OCRC) operates under similar guidelines as the EEOC and performs similar functions in Ohio that the EEOC does nationally.

OHIO CIVIL RIGHTS COMMISSION (OCRC)
220 Parsons Avenue
Columbus, Ohio 43215
Regional Office: (641) 466-5938

EXAMPLES OF SEXUAL HARASSMENT
1.   FAMILIAR OR ENDEARING NAMES
2.   TONE OF VOICE
3.   EYE CONTACT (LACK OF EYE CONTACT - STARING AT GENITALS, BREAST, ETC.)
4.   NON-VERBAL ACTIONS/INFRINGING ON PERSONAL SPACE
5.   FOLLOWING
6.   STARING
7.   TOUCHING/PATTING ON BACK OR SHOULDER
8.   CHANGING TOPIC FROM WORK RELATED MATTERS TO

PERSONAL APPEARANCE (BODY, CLOTHES, HAIR)

9. TALKING ABOUT OWN SEX LIFE

10. CAT CALLS/COMMENTS ABOUT BODY PARTS OR SEX APPEAL

11. CALENDARS AND PICTURES OF A SUGGESTIVE NATURE

12. GRABBING PARTS OF BODY

13. LEERING

14. BRUSHING AGAINST BODY

15. SEXUAL JOKES

16. MAKING THE VICTIM OR VICTIM'S PARTNER THE SUBJECT OF SEXUAL JOKES

17. WRITING ON WALLS, ELEVATORS, RESTROOMS

18. SEXUALLY EXPLICIT COMMENTS

19. LETTERS, NOTES, CARTOON OF A SUGGESTIVE NATURE, PHONE CALLS, PICTURE OF VICTIM

20. REPEATED REQUESTS FOR DATES

21. REQUESTS FOR SEXUAL FAVORS

22. ATTEMPTED RAPE

23. RAPE

CATEGORIES OF SEXUAL HARASSMENT:*

1. GENDER HARASSMENT: GENERALIZED SEXIST REMARKS AND BEHAVIOR:

2. SEDUCTIVE BEHAVIOR: INAPPROPRIATE AND OFFENSIVE, BUT ESSENTIALLY SANCTION-FREE, SEXUAL ADVANCES;

3. SEXUAL BRIBERY: SOLICITATION OF SEXUAL ACTIVITY OR OTHER SEX-LINKED BEHAVIOR BY PROMISE OF REWARDS;

4. SEXUAL COERCION: COERCION OF SEXUAL ACTIVITY BY THREAT OF PUNISHMENT; AND

5. SEXUAL ASSAULT: GROSS SEXUAL IMPOSITION, ASSAULT OR RAPE.

---

*Till, F.J. 1980 Report of Sexual Harassment: A Report on the Sexual Harassment of Students, Wash., D.C., National Advisory Council on Women's Educational Programs.

REASONS FOR NOT REPORTING SEXUAL HARASSMENT:

1. EMBARRASSMENT
2. AFRAID OF LOSING JOB/NEED THE MONEY
3. WANT TO "FIT IN" ON THE JOB/DON'T WANT TO BE SEEN AS A "TROUBLEMAKER"
4. LIKE THE JOB/DON'T WANT TO JEOPARDIZE CAREER
5. FEEL THEY WON'T BE BELIEVED/WON'T GET ANY SUPPORT
6. DON'T KNOW WHERE TO GO FOR HELP OR HOW TO FILE A COMPLAINT
7. FEEL GUILTY
8. DENIAL/TRY TO MINIMIZE SITUATION
9. AFRAID HARASSER WILL LOSE JOB
10. BELIEVE THEY CAN'T AFFORD TO FILE A COMPLAINT
11. AFRAID FOR SAFETY OF SELF AND/OR FAMILY MEMBERS
12. PREVIOUS EXPERIENCE WITH RAPE, SEXUAL ABUSE, BEING BLAMED WHEN THE VICTIM

WHY MANAGERS DON'T TAKE (PROPER) ACTION

1. DON'T TAKE SEXUAL HARASSMENT SERIOUSLY/THINK IT'S A JOKE/WOMAN IS OVERREACTING
2. THEY'RE EMBARRASSED
3. UNSURE OF HOW TO PROCEED OR HOW TO INVESTIGATE
4. THE ALLEGED HARASSER MAY BE THEIR FRIEND OR A VALUED WORKER/HAVE SENIORITY
5. MAY NOT LIKE THE INDIVIDUAL FILING THE COMPLAINT/MAY SEE THAT INDIVIDUAL AS A "PROBLEM" EMPLOYEE
6. IF IN NON-TRADITIONAL AREA FOR WOMEN - MAY NOT WANT HER IN THE JOB OR WORK SITE IN THE FIRST PLACE/FEEL SHE DESERVES OR "ASKED FOR" THE SEXUAL HARASSMENT BY BEING THERE
7. FEEL THE PROBLEM REFLECTS NEGATIVELY ON THEM OR THEIR DEPARTMENT AND WANT TO COVER IT UP

SUGGESTED ACTIONS TO TAKE AT THE WORKPLACE

1. CONFRONT THE HARASSER -- MAKE IT CLEAR YOU DO NOT WANT THIS ATTENTION
2. BEGIN A JOURNAL OR RECORD OF THE HARASSING BEHAVIOR
3. TALK TO WOMEN CO-WORKERS OR MEN CO-WORKERS
4. ASK WITNESSES TO VERIFY YOUR EXPERIENCE
5. WRITE A LETTER TO THE HARASSER (3 PARTS: STATING THE BEHAVIOR/PROBLEM, EXPLAIN YOUR REACTIONS TO IT(FEELINGS), STATE RESULTS YOU WANT - ACTIONS TO STOP, ETC.)
6. DOCUMENT YOUR OWN WORK PERFORMANCE

7.   ORGANIZE AN ACTION GROUP OR SUPPORT GROUP
     AMONG OTHER WORKERS

8.   SUBMIT A COMPLAINT IN WRITING (INCLUDING A REQUEST
     FOR ACTION) TO:

  a.   Personnel office

  b.   Union Steward or other grievance officer

  c.   EEO Officer at workplace

  d.   Affirmative Action Office

  e.   Your supervisor

  f.   The harasser's supervisor

  g.   On campus: the chairperson of the
   academic department (yours or the
   harasser's), a women's services office,
   dean of student affairs, the office of
   affirmative action

9.   KEEP COPIES OF EVERYTHING YOU SEND OR RECEIVE

...OTHER ACTIONS YOU CAN TAKE

1.   FILE A COMPLAINT WITH THE OHIO CIVIL RIGHTS
     COMMISSION (STATE)

2.   FILE A COMPLAINT WITH THE EQUAL EMPLOYMENT
     OPPORTUNITY COMMISSION (FEDERAL)

3.   FILE A COMPLAINT WITH THE BUREAU OF WORKER'S
     COMPENSATION

4.   FILE A COMPLAINT UNDER THE OCCUPATIONAL SAFETY
     AND HEALTH ACT

5.   FILE A CLAIM FOR UNEMPLOYMENT BENEFITS (IF YOU ARE

FIRED OR FORCED TO QUIT)

6.   FILE A CRIMINAL LAWSUIT (ASSAULT, BATTERY, RAPE)

7.   FILE A CIVIL LAWSUIT (BREECH OF CONTRACT,
      INTENTIONAL INFLICTION OF EMOTIONAL DURESS)

STRATEGIES FOR DEALING WITH SEXUAL HARASSMENT

I.   IDENTIFY THE RISK FACTORS

    A. Potential Harasser

        ~ insecure and easily threatened

        ~ problems with listening/interrupts

        ~ abuses power

        ~ need for control

        ~ exaggerated sense of own importance

        ~ sees women as objects/secondary importance

    B.   Work Environment

        ~ only woman

        ~ new position

        ~ non-traditional

        ~ Affirmative Action/Equal

        ~ new supervisor

II.   REDUCE THE RISK

    A. Develop positive self-esteem

    B. Approach (take self seriously, don't apologize; follow
        through)

    C. Body language

    D. Documentation of work performance

Cautionary Note: Do not assume that because a woman does not follow these suggestions she is "asking" to be sexually harassed or "deserves" to be sexually harassed, or conversely, that if a woman follows these suggestions she will be automatically protected from sexual harassment. Sexual harassment is a result of the perceptions and social and gender biases of the harasser and not the result of the behavior of the victim.

III. ASSERTIVE RESPONSE TO SEXUAL HARASSMENT

A. Name the behavior/Keep response short and to the point.

B. Negate the behavior:Say you don't like it/demand that it stops

C. Consistency in words and body language

D. Maintain your space

E. Take the situation and yourself seriously

F. Involve other people

IV. FOLLOW-UP ACTION: HOLDING THE COMPANY AND HARASSER RESPONSIBLE

A. Complaint procedures within the organization/Insist they follow the sexual harassment policy or institute such a policy if none is in place.

~ informal procedures

~ formal procedures

B. Union Grievance

C. Ohio Civil Rights Commission/EEOC

131

    D. Private law suit

    E. Criminal suit

V.   FOLLOW-UP ACTION FOR YOURSELF

    A. Support group

    B. Assertiveness class

    C. Personal counseling for stress management/reduction

    D. Self-defense class

    E. Community involvement

Take action! Do something! If sexual harassment is ignored it will become worse in most cases (about 70%). Recognize the stress it causes and the toll it takes on you personally and professionally. Do something about the sexual harassment and/or something to help yourself survive while in the situation or while fighting it.

SEXUAL HARASSMENT: AN OUTLINE FOR POLICY DEVELOPMENT AND COMPLAINT PROCEDURES

I.   ADOPT A CLEAR POLICY PROHIBITING SEXUAL HARASSMENT

This Policy should contain:

A.   A definition of sexual harassment.

B.   An explanation of the legal implications of sexual harassment.

C.   Potential personal and organizational costs of sexual harassment.

D.   Measures for swift and thorough investigation.

E.   Strong sanctions against sexual harassment which

include penalties against those who sexually harass others and penalties against managers who knowingly allow the behavior.

F.   A requirement for professional counseling for those found to have engaged in sexual harassment.

II.   SET UP COMPLAINT CHANNELS WITHIN THE ORGANIZATION

These procedures should:

A.   Be made available to all employees

B .   Insure that allegations will be taken seriously by the organization and that a fair resolution will be sought.

C.   Be as uncomplicated and streamlined as possible.

D.   Insure an action upon the complaint within a reasonable length of time.

E.   Move quickly and consistently against any employee who violates the policy.

F.   Insure confidentiality for the victim and protect her/him from any form of retaliation.

III.   PUBLICIZE THE POLICY, COMPLAINT PROCEDURES AND THE COMMITMENT OF THE ORGANIZATION.

A.   Verbally repeat the policy.

B.   Make the policy part of all new employee orientation

C.   Stress the seriousness of the policy and the

repercussions of violating it.

D.   Make sure all employees have the policy and procedures in writing.

IV.   SET UP A PREVENTION PROGRAM

Actions could include:

A.   In-service training for managers and supervisors, clarifying the issue of sexual harassment and the responsibility supervisors have for conduct in the workplace.

B.   In-service training of EEO, Affirmative Action, personnel officers, or other personnel who will be responsible for advising victims and carrying out policy.

C.   Publication of a pamphlet specifically for victims of sexual harassment which:

1.   Defines sexual harassment

2.   Lists most effective strategies and actions to stop sexual harassment.

3.   Informs individuals of their rights and the informal and formal complaint procedures within your organization.

4.   Tells what personnel are available in the organization to agist with problems associated with sexual harassment (include policy officials, counselors etc.).

5. In-service training for all staff.

V. **CLOSELY MONITOR THE SUCCESS OF THE POLICY AND COMPLAINT PROCEDURES, AND REGULARLY EVALUATE PREVENTIVE PROGRAMS**

 A. Look for signs of isolation, "freezing out", or sabotaging of an individual's work, particularly any individual who has made a complaint.

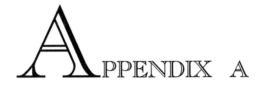

APPENDIX A

POSSIBLE
LEGAL
ACTION
CHART

Legal Remedy	Brief Description	Types of Benefits	Settlement	Problem
Title VII 1964 Civil Rights Act	Federal legislation prohibiting sex discrimination in employment; file with state and appeal through EEOC.	Monetary compensation for back pay, lost benefits and damages; possible job reinstatement.	6 months to 1 year on state level; 2-3 years federally.	Work-places with 15+ employees Must prove harassment as a form of discrimination.
Worker Compensation	Operates through State Division of Industrial Accidents. Offers benefits for injury sustained on the job.	Weekly wage benefits based on percent of income for period of disability; medical benefits.	Depends on local; nearer urban area the better; 3 to 6 with appeal taking 6 months to 1 year longer.	Usually awarded for physical Act injury; women must get medical psychiatric evaluation to be eligible for benefits; company's Insurance responsible for settlement.

Occupational Safety and Health Act	Federal Act guaranteeing a "safe and healthful work-place"; allows for inspection of work-place conditions.	Employer fined for violation responsible for correcting them.	Greatly varies	Applies to work-places with at least 15 employees.
Unemployment Insurance	Award for attributable cause for employment termination due to compelling personal	Percent of weekly salary up to a limit which varies from state to state.	Approximately 6 months.	% of women's income often too low for expense need min. length of employment; must prove attempt to change work situation by complaining to employer or requesting leave of absence

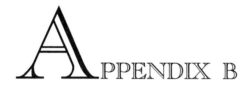

APPENDIX B

CHRONOLOGY
OF
CASE
LAW(S)

CHRONOLOGY OF CASE LAW(S) IN THE HISTORY OF SEXUAL HARASSMENT

1964 CIVIL RIGHTS ACT

Title VII of the Civil Rights Act of 1994 prohibits discrimination in employment based on sex. In general, the courts ruled on behalf of employees when a job is lost because of rejection of sexual advances, or when job benefits are lost because an employee refuses to submit to sexual advances. Further, it is considered discrimination under Title VII when a work environment has been rendered offensive as a result of sexually harassing behavior.

1972 ~ N. JAY ROGERS v. EEOC

The introduction of the "hostile work environment theory". The court acknowledged the importance of an individual's well-being and how an environment polluted with discrimination could adversely effect the psychological and emotional stability of minority group workers.

1972 ~ CONNON v. UNIVERSITY OF CHICAGO

It was the finding of the United States Supreme Court that a student had an implied right of action for protection under Title IX of Education Amendments of 1972.

1977 ~ BARNES v. COSTLE

A single event of sexual harassment may from the basis of a civil suit or an EEO complaint. The *Equal Opportunity Act o 1972* prohibits sexual harassment in federal employment and is covered by the sex discrimination provisions of the EEOC and is readdressable through the discrimination complaint procedure.

1978 ~ HEELAN v. JACKS-MANVILLS CORP.

An employer can not be held liable for harassment by a supervisor if the employer had a policy discouraging harassment; the employee failed to present the problem to a public grievance board; and the employer failed to eliminate the harassment.

1979 ~ MILLER v. BANK OF AMERICA

Even if the employer has an established policy against sexual harassment, the employer is still responsible for the sexual harassment behavior of its supervisors.

1980 EEOC GUIDELINES

EEOC incorporated sexual harassment into Guidelines on Discrimination. These Guidelines states that discrimination based on sex is prohibited, specifically determining sexual harassment a prohibited practice resulting from requests for sexual favors, unwelcomed sexual advances, verbal or physical conduct of a sexual nature when it is a condition or term of employment or when sex is used as the basis for employment decisions or creates an offensive working environment.

1980 ~ WILLIAMS v. CIVILETTI

Even if at one time, sexually advances were encouraged and/or returned, unwelcomed sexual advances as a term and condition of employment can constitute sexual harassment.

1981 ~ BUNDY v. JACKSON

Sexual harassment exists when the employer creates or condones a hostile, offensive work environment, ..."A substantially discriminatory work environment" of sexually harassing behavior or activity ... even when there is no tangible loss of job benefits.

1981 ~ EEOC v. SAGE REALTY

Determined whether employees wearing sexually provocative clothing as a condition of employment is a violation of Title VII and the sexual harassment guidelines.

1981 WRIGHT v. METHODIST YOUTH SERVICES

Determines that unwelcomed sexual advances are prohibited under Title VII even if the parties involved are of the same sex.

1982 ~ COLEY v. CONSOLIDATED RAIL CORP.

Determined that resignation be considered as an employer termination if the employee resigned as a result of an intolerable work environment created by discrimination of other unlawful acts that would compel a *reasonable person* to resign.

1982 ~ GAN v. KEPRO CIRCUIT SYSTEMS

Court ruling: a female employee who regularly engages in vulgar language, asked male employees about their sex lives, discussed her own marital sexual relations... was not constructively discharged. Further that this behavior helps to create an adverse work environment and in fact welcomes the conduct of sexual harassment.

1983 ~ KATZ v. DOLE

An employer is liable when he/she fails to respond to acts of sexual harassment. The employer is responsible for acts of sexual harassment on the part of supervisors or co-workers. Indicating the existence of a policy against sexual harassment does not constitute an adequate response. Court noted that sexual harassment was in fact "an intentional assault on an individual's innermost privacy."

1983 ~ CUMMINGS v. WALSH CONSTRUCTION CO.

A female employee rejected the sexual advances of superiors and was retaliated against and required to perform harsh and menial tasks. Even though the company had a policy, they were liable for the activity because top level personnel was involved and had knowledge of the hostile work environment.

1984 ~ BARRETT v. OMAHA NATIONAL BANK

An employer is not liable for events of sexual harassment by co-workers when the employer promptly responds to the complaint of sexual harassment by... conducting a full investigation, implement measures to stop the behavior and indicate disciplinary action should the harassment continues.

1985 ~ STATE OF NEW YORK v. HAMILTON

Employer is liable for sexual harassment conduct by its contractors, customers, or other non-employees when the employer is aware of the conduct and is in a position to control the conduct but fails to take appropriate and immediate action.

1985 ~ HORN v. DUKE HOMES

A plant supervisor used his authority to hire and fire employees based on the employees consent to have sex in exchange for keeping their jobs. The Company was held liable under the doctrine of *respondeat superior.*

1985 ~ HAYES LIVING HEALTH CARE AGENCY

The court ruled that an employee was sexually harassed when her superior invited her into his hotel room, offering wine, pornographic movies and magazines and attempt to restrain her departure.

1986 ~ MERITOR SAVINGS BANK v. VINSON

Further Court ruling determined that how a victim dresses, talks, or behaves can only be considered when those factors are relevant to whether or not the sexual behavior is question was welcomed or unwelcomed. Although an employer is not automatically liable for every harassing act by a supervisor or manager, failure of an employee to notify the employer does not necessarily relieve the employer of the responsibilities regarding sexual harassment.

1986 ~ SCOTT v. SEARS, ROEBUCK & CO.

An employee is liable for the harassing behavior of its employees under EEOC Guidelines "where the employer knows or should have known of the conduct, unless it can be shown that it took immediate and appropriate corrective action."

1987 ~ SHAW v. NEBRASKA DEPARTMENT OF CORRECTIONAL SERVICES

When males of the promotion selection committee used the terms, *girls, dear, and honey,* a "sexist" environment was created for the females those terms were used to address.

1988 ~ LEWELLYN v. CELANESE CORP.

When a female employee was forced to quite her job as a truck driver because she received sexual solicitations and threats from her co-workers, to the point of resignation, the court ruled that she had been "constructively discharged" and equated this an illegal firing.

1988 ~ BENNETT v. CORROON & BLACK CORP.

A female employee charged that she was being sexually harassed through the depiction of sexually explicit cartoon characters in the men's rest room. The court defined these actions as sexual harassment, but the alleged victim was not awarded damages because management took corrective measures and continued to pay the employer until she found other employment.

1990 ~ KING v. BOARD OF REGENTS UNIVERSITY OF WISCONSIN

The courts ruled that sexual harassment of public employees may be in violation of the Equal Protection Clause of the Fourteenth Amendment.

1991 ~ ROBINSON v. JACKSONVILLE SHIPYARDS

Nude pin-ups in a workplace were found to constitute sexual harassment particularly when a "reasonably woman" would find the environment offensive and abusive.

1992 ~ FRANKLIN v. GWINNETT COUNTY

The Court ruled that students can be awarded monetary damages and other remedies when they sue a school or school officials for sexual harassment.

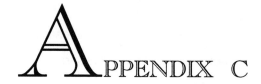

APPENDIX C

GLOSSARY
OF
TERMS

Glossary of Terms With Reference To Sexual Harassment

Compensatory Damages

Actual financial losses; The calculated dollar amount awarded to complainants to make them whole and/or return them to the position they would have been in prior to the act of discrimination.

Constructive Discharge

When an employee is forced to resign because of intolerable terms and conditions of employment, resignation can be treated as a dismissal.

Constructive Notice

An implied notice, wherein, under existing conditions, an employee should have known sexual harassment exits.

Hostile Work Environment

Unwelcome sexual conduct that creates an offensive, hostile, or intimidating working environment.

Inter-Cultural Sexual Harassment

Unwelcome sexual conduct that creates an offensive, intimidating, and/or hostile enviornment between two-like groups, i.e., race, gender, religion, etc.

Negligent Retention

An employer's failure to remove an individual who can cause foreseeable harm to others.

Non-Verbal Harassment

Sexual suggestive acts of a non-verbal nature; i.e. pornographic pictures, drawings, unwanted gifts, cards, or letters, leering, etc.

Physical Harassment

Touching oneself or another person in a sexually suggestive manner.

Punitive Damages

A specific dollar amount awarded to victim to punish the defendant's conduct of sexual harassment and to deter potential offenses.

Quid Pro Quo

Something for something. Unwelcome acts of a sexual nature in exchange for employment benefits; or the loss of employment benefits due to the rejection of unwelcome acts of a sexual nature.

Reasonable Person

Responding the way a "reasonable person" would under like circumstances. A standard of behavior.

Respondeat Superior Liability

Wherein, the employer is liable for acts of sexual harassment of a supervisor.

Sexual Harassment (1980 EEOC)

Unwelcome sexual advances, requests for sexual favors, and other verbal, or physical conduct of a sexual nature constitute sexual harassment when 1) submission to such conduct is made either explicitly or implicitly a term or condition of an individual's employment, 2) submission to or rejection of such conduct by an individual is used as a basis for employment decisions affecting such individual, or 3) such conduct has the purpose or effect of unreasonably interfering with an individual's work performance or creating an intimidating, hostile, or offensive work enviornment.

Verbal Harassment

Sexual comments; i.e., sexual jokes, riddles, stories, and or making sexual statements about another individual.

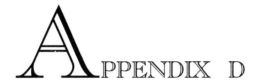

APPENDIX D

BLACK ON BLACK
SEXUAL HARASSMENT
QUESTIONNAIRE
GRAPHIC
RESULTS

A questionnaire was circulated throughout the Afrikan American Community. Afrikan American organizations and agencies, as well as individuals participated. The questionnaire requested the participants to provide honest responses to a series of questions regarding sexual harassment. Participants were informed that their answers were confidential and would be used to create educational tools to help prevent sexual harassment.

Participants were given this definition of sexual harassment:

Repeated or deliberate verbal, non-verbal, and/or physical behavior of a sexual nature that is unwelcomed. e.g. unwanted sexual jokes, suggestions, comments and/or pressure for sexual favors; suggestive looks; leering; squeezes or touches; or repeatedly brushing against someone's body. SEXUAL HARASSMENT is an "unlawful employment practice" under Title VII of the 1964 Civil Rights Act and is a form of sex discrimination.

Participants ranged from age 16 to 66 years old. Participants were both Afrikan American males and females.

Participants occupation(s) were varied and included:

Youth Counselor(s), Member of the United States Army, Finance & Development Professional, Regional Manager, Facilitators, Telemarketer, Social Worker(s), Attorneys, Banker, Consultants, Students, Self-employed Individuals, Individuals in Management, Unemployed Individuals, Secretaries, Account Clerk,

Homemakers, Systems Analysts, Health Care Providers, Prevention Educators, Rehabilitations & Correction Personnel, Program Coordinators, Cashier, Human Resource Professionals, Administrative Assistants, Retired Individuals, Engineers, Nursing, Upholstery Professional.

Participants were asked if they were heterosexual, homosexual, or bi-sexual.

Approximately 90% responded that they were heterosexual, 2% stated that they were homosexual or bi-sexual, and 8% did not respond to this inquiry.

Participants were asked the following question:

~ Have you ever felt that you have been sexually harassed?

~ Do you know someone who has been a victim of sexual harassment?

~ Do you know some one who sexually harasses other people?

~ Have you ever harassed other people?

~ Is/was your harasser someone you work for/with?

~ Is/was your sexual harasser a family member?

~ Were/are you able to tell your harasser to stop harassing you?

~ Would you speak up in the future if you experienced sexual harassment again?

~ Do you feel people who complain about sexual harassment are just too sensitive?

~ Are you in litigation?

~ Did you have sex with your harasser?

~ What race group did your harasser belong to?

Key to graphs: Two shaded graphs are the collective results of total participants (both male and female).

Multi-shaded graphs are the results of the same participants, however, answers are identified by gender.

Have you ever felt that you have been sexually harassed?

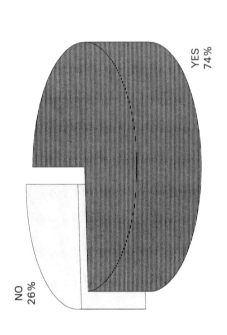

YES
74%

NO
26%

YES

NO

Have you ever felt that you have been sexually harassed?

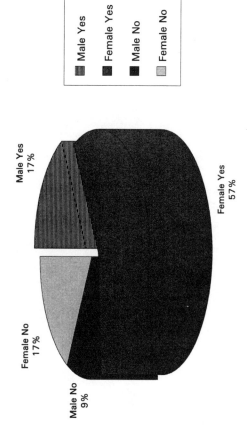

Male Yes
17%

Female No
17%

Male No
9%

Female Yes
57%

Male Yes
Female Yes
Male No
Female No

Do you know someone who has been a victim of sexual harassment?

YES

NO

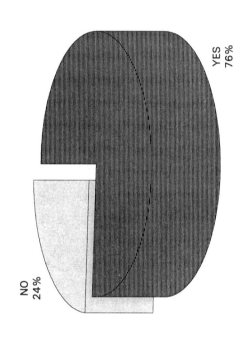

NO
24%

YES
76%

Do you know someone else who has been the victim of sexual harassment?

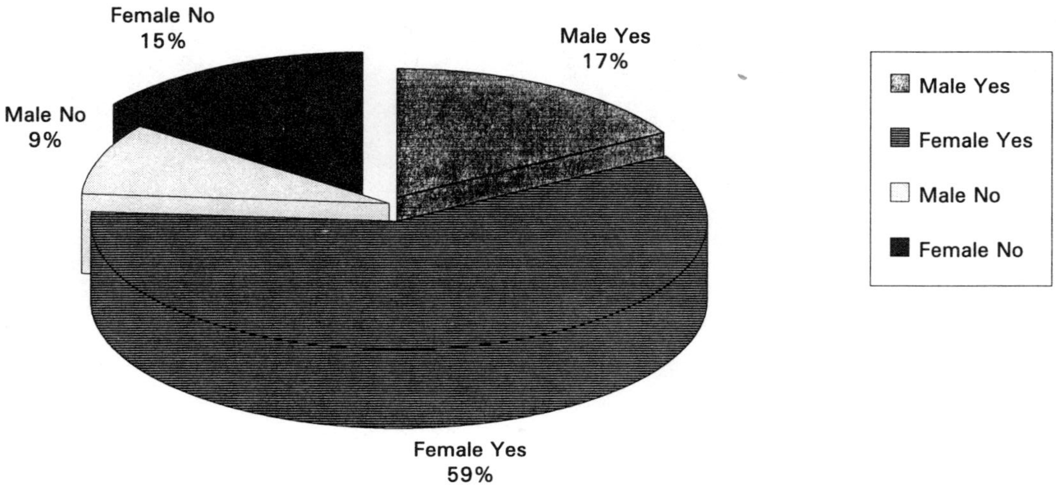

Male Yes
17%

Female Yes
59%

Female No
15%

Male No
9%

Legend:
- Male Yes
- Female Yes
- Male No
- Female No

Do you know someone who sexually harasses other people?

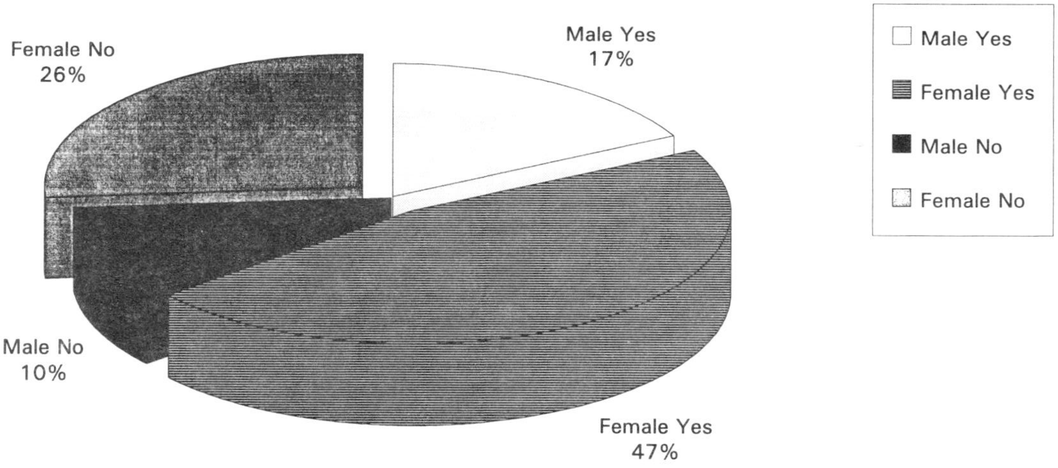

Male Yes
17%

Female Yes
47%

Female No
26%

Male No
10%

Legend:
- Male Yes
- Female Yes
- Male No
- Female No

Have you ever sexually harassed someone?

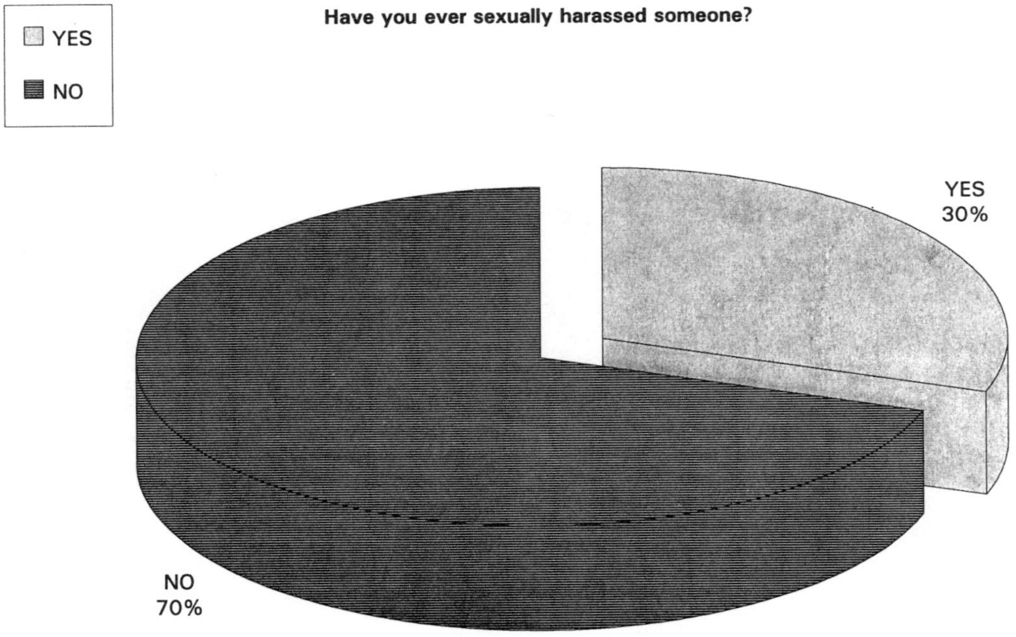

YES
30%

NO
70%

YES

NO

Have you ever sexually harassed someone?

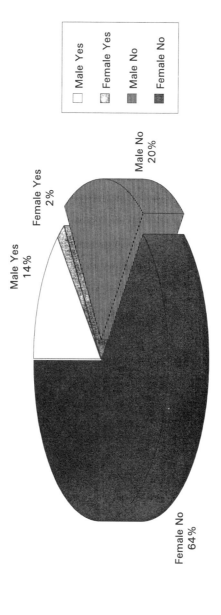

Male Yes
14%

Female Yes
2%

Male No
20%

Female No
64%

- Male Yes
- Female Yes
- Male No
- Female No

Is/was your sexual harasser someone you work for/with?

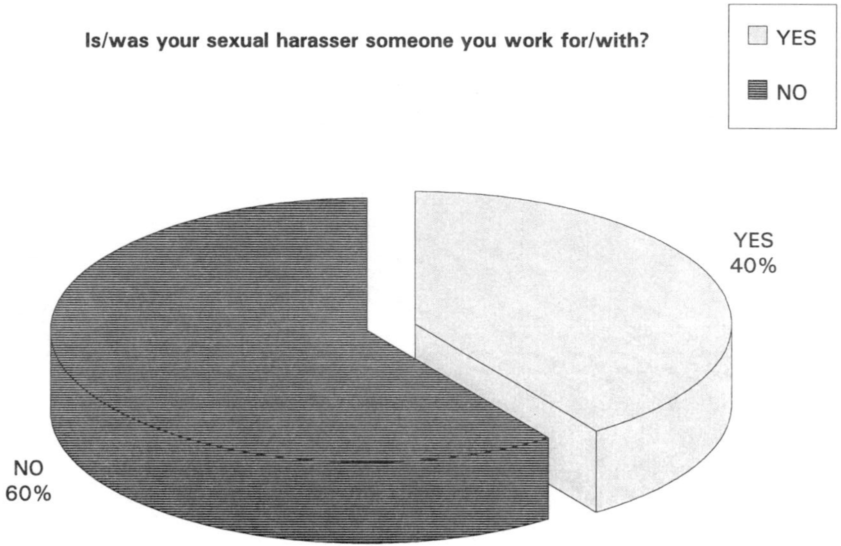

YES
NO

YES
40%

NO
60%

Is/was your sexual harasser someone you work for/with?

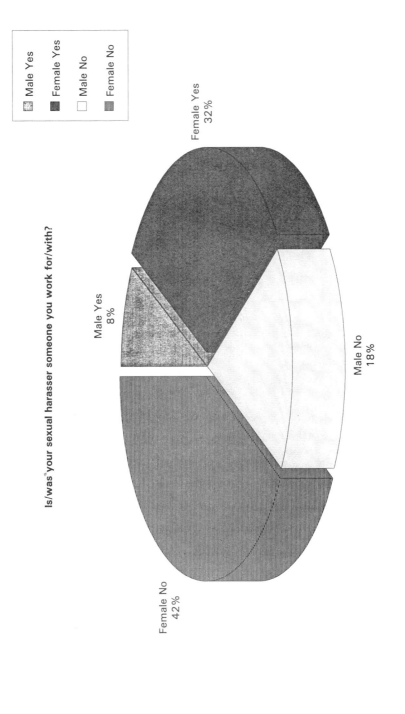

Male Yes
8%

Female Yes
32%

Male No
18%

Female No
42%

Male Yes
Female Yes
Male No
Female No

Is/was your harasser a family member?

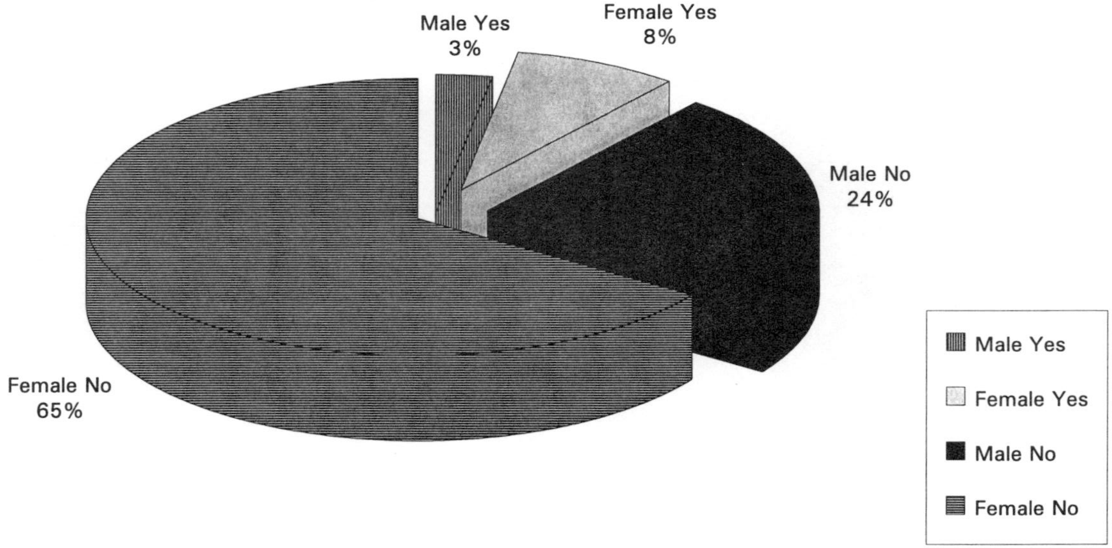

Male Yes 3%

Female Yes 8%

Male No 24%

Female No 65%

Legend:
- Male Yes
- Female Yes
- Male No
- Female No

Is/was your sexual harasser a family member?

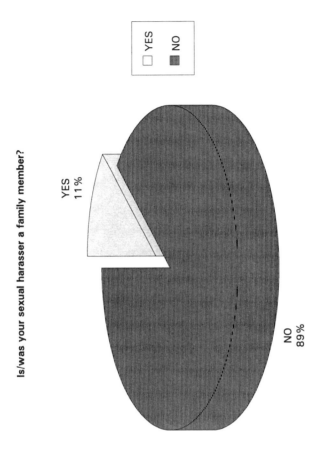

YES
11%

NO
89%

YES
NO

Were/are you able to tell your harasser to stop harassing you?

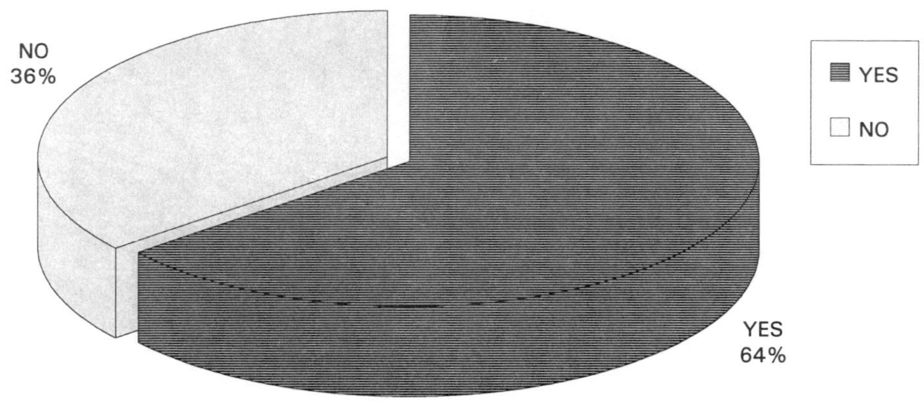

YES
64%

NO
36%

■ YES
□ NO

Were/are you able to tell your harasser to stop harassing you?

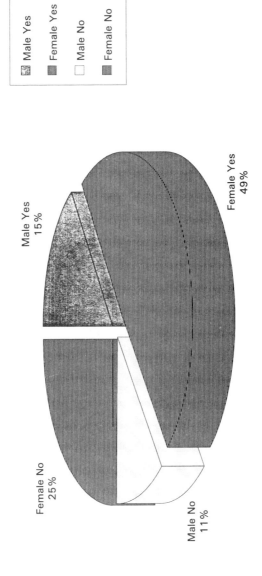

Male Yes
15%

Female Yes
49%

Female No
25%

Male No
11%

Male Yes
Female Yes
Male No
Female No

Would you speak up in the future if you experienced sexual harassment again?

YES
NO

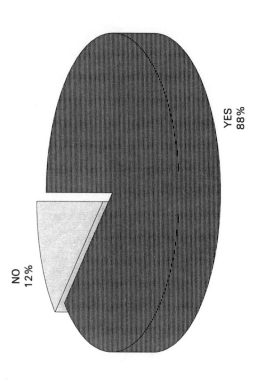

NO
12%

YES
88%

Would you speak up in the future if you experienced sexual harasssment again?

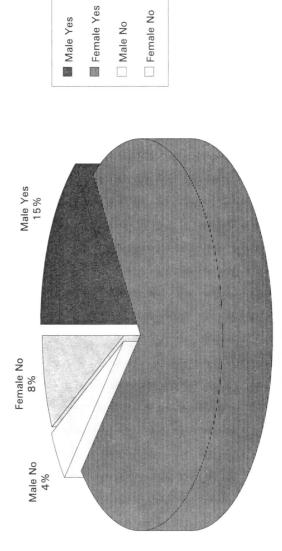

Male Yes
15%

Female No
8%

Male No
4%

Female Yes
73%

- Male Yes
- Female Yes
- Male No
- Female No

Do you feel that people who complain about sexual harassment are just too sensitive?

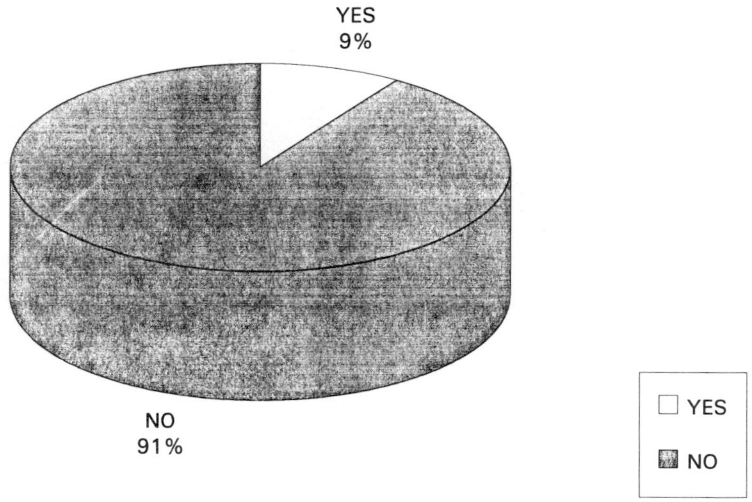

YES
9%

NO
91%

☐ YES

▩ NO

Are you currently in litigation?

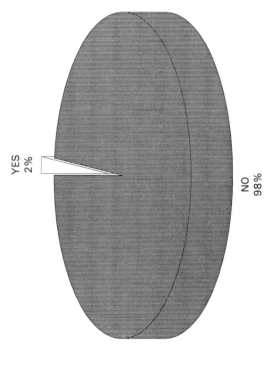

YES
2%

NO
98%

☐ YES

▤ NO

Did you have sex with your harasser?

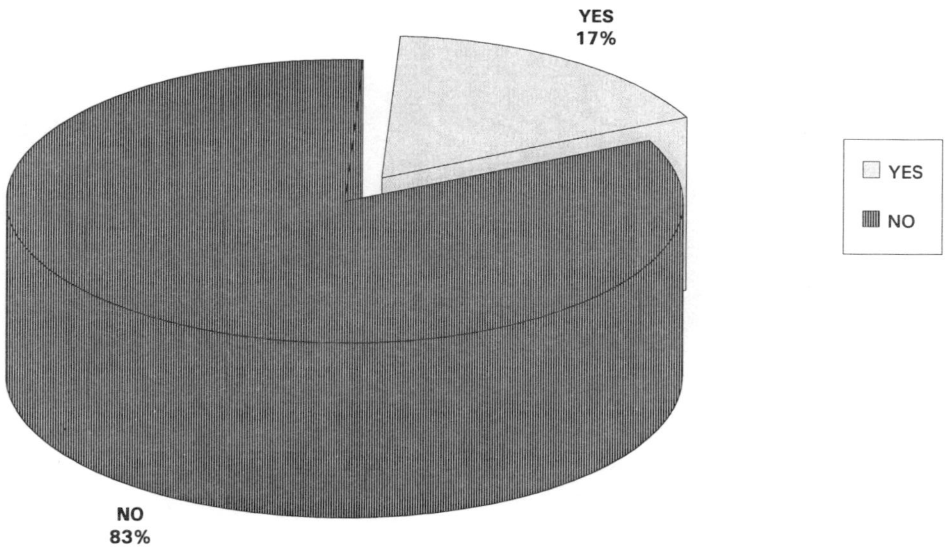

YES
17%

NO
83%

YES
NO

Black Females were asked, "What race group did your harasser belong to?"

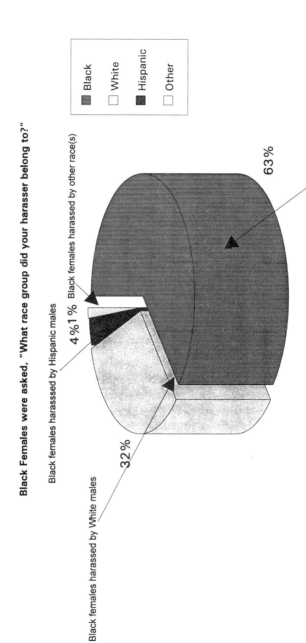

	Black
	White
	Hispanic
	Other

Black females harasssed by Hispanic males

4%1% Black females harassed by other race(s)

Black females harassed by White males

32%

63%

Black females were harassed by Black males by over 60%

Black males were asked, "What race group did your harasser belong to?"

Black males harassed by other race(s) 0%

Black males harassed by Hispanic females

4%

Black males harassed by white females

29%

67%

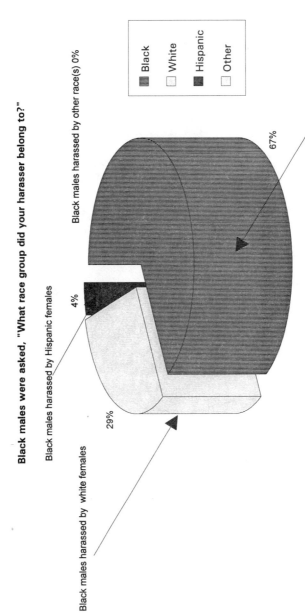

Legend:
- Black
- White
- Hispanic
- Other

Black males were harassed by Black females by over 67%

Have you ever felt that you
have been sexually
harassed?

The same individuals were asked:

How did being sexually harassed make you feel?

Some of the descriptives of how they felt included:

Stressed	Nervous	Helpless	Ugly
Worried	Angry	Sexy	Trapped
Good	Pressured	Victimized	Happy
Dirty	Depressed	Upset	Wanted
Attractive	Needed		

Note: Some of the respondents, even though they stated that they felt stressed, nervous, and pressured, they also said they felt wanted, sexy, attractive and/or needed, even good.

When asked: If you are/were a victim of sexual harassment, do/did you suffer from any physical symptoms because of this experience? A very large percentage said they experienced physical symptoms.

Some of the symptoms included:

Anxiety	Seizure	Headaches	Forgetfulness
Fatigue	Sleepiness	Tension	Lost appetite
Nausea	Dizziness	Diarrhea	Increased appetite
Cramps	Nervousness	Depression	Yeast infection

Participants were asked if they sexually harassed others, how it made them feel? Their response:

Popular	Strong	Slick	Depressed
Flirtatious	Powerful	Good	Handsome
Fun	Sexy	Important	

Some participants provided written comments:

...being sexually harassed made me feel completely nasty.

...I never have sexually harassed others and never will.

...I quit my job at places I was being sexually harassed.

...On the job, how you carry yourself - you get respect.

...the emotion I felt was one of uncertainty.

...even though he forced me, I ended up liking it and kept my job.

...I was not aware of the harassment.

...I feel as if I am being prevented from making a choice.

...I have not sexually harassed anyone.

...after I did my work as a contractor, my harasser tried to pressure me into a relationship for payment.

...I would only feel trapped depending on the harasser.

...I have never been sexually harassed so I can't comment on how it makes me feel.

...I always don't think it's sexual harassment. Sometimes it's just flirting.

...my uncle introduced me to homosexuality.

...I am not sure it's sexual harassment, but more of a come-on.

...because I am a male, I was not suppose to say, "No".

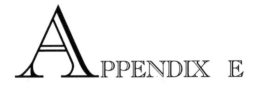

APPENDIX E

AGENCY
&
RESOURCE
LIST

ALABAMA
EEOC
Birmingham District
Office
1900 Third Avenue,
North Suite 101
Birmingham, AL
35203
(205) 731-0082

ARIZONA
EEOC
Phoenix District
Office
4520 North Central
Avenue
Suite 300
Phoenix, AZ 85012
(602) 640-5000

ARKANSAS
EEOC
Little Rock Area
Office
320 West Capitol
Avenue
Suite 621
Little Rock, AR
72201
(501) 324-5060

CALIFORNIA
EEOC
Los Angeles District
Office
3660 Wilshire
Boulevard Fifth Flr
Los Angeles, CA
90010
(213) 251-7278

EEOC
Oakland Local
Office
1333 Broadway

Room 430
Oakland, CA 94612
(415)273-7588

EEOC
880 Front Street
Room 45-21
San Diego, CA
92188
(619) 557-6288

EEOC
San Francisco
District
901 Market Street
Suite 500
San Francisco, CA
94103
(415) 744-6500

Equal Rights
Advocates
1663 Mission St
Suite 550
San Francisco, CA
94103
(415) 621-0505
*Legal counseling &
advice in
Spanish & English*

COLORADO
EEOC
Denver District
Office
1845 Sherman St
Second Floor
Denver, CO 80203
(303 866-1300

FLORIDA
EEOC
Miami District Office
1 Northeast First St
Sixth Floor

Miami, FL 33132
(305) 536-4491

EEOC
Tampa Area Office
Timberlake Fed.
Bldg
501 East Polk Street
Suite 1020
Tampa, FL 33602
(813) 228-2310

GEORGIA
EEOC
Atlanta District
Office
75 Piedmont
Avenue NE
Suite 1100
Atlanta, GA 30335
(404) 331-6093

HAWAII
EEOC
Honolulu Local
Office
677 Ala Moana Blvd.
Suite 404
Honolulu, HI 96813
(808) 541-3120

ILLINOIS
EEOC
Chicago District
Office
536 South Clark St
Room 930
Chicago, IL 60605
(312) 353-2713

American Bar
Association
Commission on
Women in the
Profession

177

750 North Lake Shore Drive
Chicago, IL 60611
(312) 988-5668

INDIANA
EEOC
Indianapolis District Office
46 East Ohio Street
Room 456
Indianapolis, IN 46204
(317) 226-7212

IOWA
National Conference of State Legislatures
Women's Network
1607 250th Avenue
Corwith, IA 50430
(515) 583-2156

KENTUCKY
EEOC
Louisville Area Office
600 Martin Luther King, Jr. Place,
Room 268
Louisville, KY 40202
(502)582-6082

LOUISIANA
EEOC
New Orleans District Office
701 Lyola Avenue
Suite 600
New Orleans, LA 70113
(504)589-2329

MARYLAND
EEOC

Baltimore District Office
111 Market Place
Suite 4000
Baltimore, MD 21202
(301)962-3932

MASSACHUSETTS
EEOC
Boston Area Office
1 Congress Street
Room 1001
Boston, MA 02114

MICHIGAN
EEOC
Detroit District Office
477 Michigan Ave
Room 1540
Detroit, MI 48226
(313) 226-7636

MINNESOTA
EEOC
Minneapolis Local Office
220 Second Street S
Room 108
Minneapolis, MN 55401
(612) 370-3330

MISSISSIPPI
EEOC
Jackson Area Office
Cross Road Bldg.
Complex
207 West Amite St
Jackson, MS 39201
(601) 965-4537

MISSOURI
EEOC
Kansas City Area

Office
911 Walnut Street
Tenth Floor
Kansas City, MO 64106
(816) 426-5773

EEOC
St. Louis District Office
625 North Euclid St
Fifth Floor
St. Louis, MO 63108
(314) 425-6585

NEW JERSEY
EEOC
Newark Area Office
60 Park Place
Room 301
Newark, NJ 07102
(201) 645-63383

NEW MEXICO
EEOC
Albuquerque Area Office
505 Marquette, NW
Suite 1105
Albuquerque, NM 87102-2189

NEW YORK
EEOC
Buffalo Local Office
28 Church Street
Room 301
Buffalo, NY 14202
(716) 846-4441

EEOC
New York District Office
90 Church Street
Room 1501

New York, NY
10007
(212) 264-7161

Amer. Civil Liberties
Union Women's
Rights Project
132 West 43rd St
New York, NY
10036
(212) 944-9800

N.A.A.C.P. Legal
Defense and
Educational Fund
99 Hudson Street
New York, NY
10013
(212) 219-1900

Ms. Foundation for
Women Ad Hoc
Sexual Harassment
Coalition
141 Fifth Avenue
New York, NY
10010
(212) 353-8580

NOW Legal Defense
Fund
National Association
of Women & the Law
99 Hudson Street
12th Floor
New York, NY
10013
(212) 925-6635

Coalition of Labor
Union Women
15 Union Square
New York, NY
10003
(212) 242-07000

National Council on
Research for
Women
The Sara Delano
Roosevelt
Memorial House
47-49 East 65th St
New York, NY
10021
(212) 570-5001

NORTH CAROLINA
EEOC
Greensboro Local
Office
324 West Market St
Room 27
P.O. Box 3363
Greensboro, NC
27401
(919) 333-5174

EEOC
Charlotte District
Office
5500 Central
Avenue
Charlotte, NC 28212
(704) 567-7100

EEOC
1309 Annapolis
Drive
Raleigh, NC 27608
(919) 856-44064

OHIO
EEOC
Cincinnati Area
Office
The Ameritrust
Building
525 Vine Street
Suite 810
Cincinnati, OH

45202
(513) 684-2851

EEOC
Cleveland District
Office
1375 Euclid Avenue
Room 600
Cleveland, OH
44115
(216) 522-2001

Ohio Civil Rights
Commission -
Central Office
220 Parsons Ave
Columbus, OH
43215
(614) 466-5938

Cleveland Regional
Office
Frank Lausche Bldg
885
615 W. Superior Ave
Cleveland, OH
44113
(216) 787-3150

Toledo Regional
Office
One Government Ctr
936 Jackson &
Erie Streets
Toledo, OH 43604
(419) 245-2900

Cincinnati Regional
Office
Goodall Complex
Suite 200
324 West 9th Street
Cincinnati, OH
45202
(513) 852-3344

Akron Regional
Office
Akron Government
Bldg. Suite 205
161 South High St
Akron, OH 44308
(216) 379-3100

Dayton Regional
Office
Miami Valley Tower
Suite 800
40 West 4th Street
Dayton, OH 45402
(513) 285-6500

Women Against
Sexual Harassment
W.A.S.H.
616 Five Oaks Ave.
Dayton, OH 45406
(513) 274-2273

Treasure Associates
P.O. Box 14301
Dayton, OH 45413
(513) 339-9965

National Association
of Working Women:
9 to 5
1224 Hudson Road
Cleveland, OH
44113
(216) 566-9308

Committee Against
Sexual Harassment
YWCA
65 S. Fourth Street
Columbus, Ohio
43215

OKLAHOMA
EEOC

Oklahoma City Area
Office
531 Couch Drive
Oklahoma City, OK
73102
(405)231-4911

PENNSYLVANIA
EEOC
Pittsburgh Area
Office
1000 Liberty Avenue
Room 2038-A
Pittsburgh, PA
15222
(412) 644-3444

EEOC
Philadelphia District
Office
1421 Cherry Street
Tenth Floor
Philadelphia, PA
19102
(215) 656-7020

SOUTH CAROLINA
EEOC
Greenville Local
Office
15 South Main St
Suite 530
Greenville, SC
29601
(803) 241-4400

TENNESSEE
EEOC
Memphis District
Office
1407 Union Avenue
Suite 621
Memphis, TN 38104
(901) 722-2617

EEOC
Nashville Area
Office
50 Vantage Way
Suite 202
Nashville, TN 37228
(615) 736-5820

TEXAS
EEOC
Dallas District Office
8303 Elmbrook Dr
Dallas, TX 75247
(214) 767-7015

EEOC
Houston District
Office
1919 Smith Street
Seventh Floor
Houston, TX 77002
(713) 653-3320

EEOC
San Antonio District
Office
5410 Federicksburg
Road Suite 200
San Antonio, TX
78229

VIRGINIA
EEOC
Norfolk Area Office
252 Monticello Ave
First Floor
Norfolk, VA 23510
(804) 441-3470

EEOC
Richmond Area
Office
3600 W. Broad St.
Room 229
Richmond, VA

23230
(804) 771-2692

**WASHINGTON,
D.C.**
EEOC
Washington Field
Office
1400 L Street N.W.
Suite 200
Washington, D.C.
20005
(202) 272-7377

Federally Employed
Women Legal and
Education Fund
1400 Eye St. NW
Washington, D.C.
20005
(202) 462-5253

Mexican American
Legal Defense Fund
1430 K Street, NW
Washington, D.C.
20005
(202) 628-4074

WISCONSIN
EEOC
Milwaukee District Office
310 W. Wisconsin Avenue
Suite 800
Milwaukee, WI 53203
(414) 297-1111

*D*ear:
Arthur, Kevin, Ali, Gary, Jomo, Lamont, Douglas, James, Bob, Joe, Eric, Walter, Ralph, Derrick, LoRin, Keith, King, Leonard, Dave, Bill, John, Khris, Rodney, Sam, Mike, Charles, Phil, Jeff, Ellis, Richard, Bart, Willie, Paul, Dog, Pimpdaddy, Roger, Dale, Lenny, Buster, Theo, Tommy, Anthony, Tony, Jerry, Karl, Dorian, Lamar, Robert, Bobby, Fishbone, Marvin, Lawrence, Matthew, Psycho, Martin, Christopher, James, Eddie, Ronald, Alvin, Raymar, Sonny, Albert, Saul, Terry, Reggie, Aaron, Ernest, Clarence, Ted, Eugene, MacDaddy, Calvin, London, Arnold, Malik, Pedro, Wesley, Leon, Danny, Larry, Malcom, Adam, Luther, Marcus, Edward, Kenny, Brandon, Joshua, Ray, Carlos, Louis, Nathan, Shortdog, Jonathan, Blair, Chaka, Issiah, Domonic, Sugardaddy, Darryl, Len, Harold, Jack, Jessie, Donald, Huey, Bobby, Shooter, Muhammad, Bernie, Ivory, Maurice, Andre, Money, Andrew, Jarman, Fred, Bo, Randy, Spike, Booker, Alexander, Alonzo, T-Bird, August, Terrence, Abraham, Clyde, Stanley, Craig, Royce, Elijah, Cornell, Romone, Weldon, Blain, Duckman, Willis, Dick, Radar, Shawn, Rasheed, Peter, Wallace, Black, Byron, Samaj, Monster, George, Barry, G-Money, Nelson, Player, Ashe', Jordon, Jacob, Oliver, Lee, Henry, Ernest, T-Bone, LeRoy, Killer, Bryant, Chuck, Les, Gordon, Jacque, Kareem, Bradford, Jazz, Calvin, Trey, Otis, Wilson, Mello, Dudley, Omari, Stephan, Walkili, Jerad, Kid Frost, Abraham, Ajamu', Walli, Slybird, Candyman, Poochie, Demitrius, Dexter, Garland, Smitty, Tupak, Harpo, Junebug, Patrick, Miller, Quincy, Rowan, Squig, Cleveland, Reginald, Kenyan, Joseph, Spencer, Victor, Scarface, Greg, Cashdollar, Jimmi Lee, Lefty, Cain, Twigman, Olson, Carson, Ingram, Bently, O'Dog, Red, Cleophus, Juice, Donald, Evans, Leo, Joel, Dotson, Joey, Hubert, Earthquake, Jason, Glenn, Bebop, Diamond, Duncan, Franklin, Sugarfoot, Gilbert, Booker, Atiba, Tobie, Ruben, Kyle, Man, JoJo, Bobby, General, Elton, Horace, Garfield, Dolamite, Oliver, Lorenzo, Big Daddy, Chaney, Todd, Arnold, Lucas, Wilt, Gene, Ace, Clifford, Nino, Clay, Ross, Bennie, T-Tee, Scott, Shortdog, Vic, Cal, Easy, Carlton, Yellow Dog, Cook, Woody, Wink, Fisher,

Roy, Littleman, Roth, Skillet, Stedman, Dwight, Roosevelt, Jeremy, Footy, Jan, Pimpdaddy, Money, Lance, Chester, Star, Cash, Shaft, Scotty, Topper, Benson, Wyndle, Woody, Murphy, Norman, Homes.... and all other brothers unnamed:

I hope you have read this book with much attention so that you could see, feel, and hear the cry of your sisters. There's a peculiar pain penetrating the hearts of thousands of your Afrikan American women. Your mothers, your sisters, your wives, and your daughters are suffering! We are hurting and we are crying. *Some* of you refuse to see our tears and you ignore our unbearable pain. WHY? Why are we being hurt and abandoned by so many of you? Too many of you?

As your spiritual and cultural sisters, and as the womb that gave you birth, we have a right to know. We have a duty to tell you that you are hurting us; point out to you how you are hurting us and tell you why you must stop!

The ways that you cause us such internal pain are many. You write songs about us and call us bitches, "ho's", and God knows what else. You father our children, then some of you refuse to help rear them. You choose to kill and maim one another as animals for principles that are evil and destructive. Instead of helping one another as brothers, and you end up either dead or locked up. *Where is the love?*

You trade-in the ethics of your true manhood in exchange for mental and lacivious games with white girls as you permit them to lobotomize your mind through the oral manipulation of your own penis -- resulting in the castration of your own race. You put dope in your veins and in the veins of your women and children so that you can drive around in a fancy car, live in a fancy house, and sport gold teeth. Need we say more?

This book is about a short laundry list of what needs to be fixed now and what can and must be fixed now. There's not enough space and time within its covers to capture our entire dilemma. Your strained relationship with your mother, your cultural sisters, your wives and your daughters did not happen overnight, and some things will take a little more time to heal than they did to inflict. However, there are many things that we can do now to help each other move closer toward our long- overdue healing. All it will cost us is a good, long, honest and individual look in the mirror and a desire for an individual commitment to positive change.

This book is about Black on Black Sexual Harassment. Brothers harassing sisters. Don't miss out on the message by trying to debate whether sexual harassment exists in other combinations. It does. That's another book, perhaps the one you should write. Hopefully, this book will encourage you to write it so that we can help each other. The responsibility for change lies with both of us.

Many of you are victimizing us in our homes, in the workplace, in school hallways, on college campuses, and/or on the streets, and it has to stop. I have found through personal and vicarious experiences, that too many Black women suffer daily from this act of gross disrespect. The internal conflict that Black on Black sexual harassment creates, leaves a bitter taste with deep feelings of anguish and disappointment. The anguish turns into anger and, eventually, the disappointment turns into a strong sense of duty; a duty to speak up and out against someone we feel should be our protector. Speaking out for many of us creates a peculiar kind of pain.

Not only is sexual harassment illegal and immoral, it violates our spiritual nature and erodes our cultural bond. It separates our souls and prevents us from unifying our efforts. An Afrikan man spiritually aligned with his Afrikan woman creates power; power that releases an non-penetratable healing balm; power that builds minds, nations, and causes the universe to unveil her mysteries. Remember Khamit? When we violate our spiritual bond, we curse our very existence.

Brothers, when you harass us, you glorify your false sense of superiority and allow your thoughts, feelings, words, actions, and reactions to be controlled by lascivious spirits. You operate out of darkness abandoning your light of wisdom. You fail to see the internal damage you bring first to yourself and second, to your victim, your sister, who is the nurturer of your seed and the teacher of your community.

Often your sisters internalize their anguish and begin to think as captives in bondage to a slave master. They begin to move out of fear; feeling helpless and overwhelmed. They become so preoccupied with their own pain that it blinds them and they may in turn inflict pain upon you as a defense.

Brothers, like you, we too are trapped, failing to find the inner strength to free ourselves. Can't you see that together we hold the key to free one another. Instead of riding the self-blaming, volunteer victim's merry-go-round, one vicious cycle after, and pointing a blaming finger at one another, let us hold each others hand. Let us at least try again. Let us look for reasons why we must succeed at uniting instead of embracing vapors of excuses that build monuments to nothingness.

Many of you occupy positions of authority; positions that our ancestral parents only dreamed of; positions that have taken us out of the cotton field and into the fields of politics, technology, education, entertainment, medicine, and science. When you forget whose sacrificial shoulders you stand on and whose spilled blood we all live by, you forget your moral obligation to one another. You forget from whence you came and what it took to overcome the moral suffering we so long endured. You tend to deny the importance of staying spiritually in tune and forget that you **are** your sisters keeper, not her stumbling block. Brothers, if we can't turn to you, where can we go?

185

The Black woman has suffered a peculiar kind of pain for centuries by carrying her weight and the weight of her people. Lest we forget brothers, that we were both once considered a personal piece of property- *chattel.* When you were bent over in the cotton fields, we were right there beside you. When you worked from sun up to sun down on the rice and sugar plantations, we were there too, toiling the same long humiliating hours; bearing your pain *and* the pain of our children. Remember? We're both descendants of the largest holocaust in the recorded history of mankind. We've both survived the diabolical whims of our slave masters. Let's not subject one another to that again. We need to ask God to search out our hearts and minds and renew in us a spirit of brotherhood and sisterhood, but most of all, self-love.

Black man, we need you to stand up by our sides and be counted as men. We need you to be our helpmates in the workplace not our taskmasters. Like you, and too many times because of you, we are heads of households and have a right to earn a living without humiliation and pain -- at least not from one another. One more note brothers. Even if you're not the one harassing us, but you know a brother who does and you keep silent, you are just as guilty. You have a spiritual, cultural, and moral obligation to pull that brother aside and strongly admonish him and remind him of his true manhood and heritage.

And, if you are uncertain if your words, action, or non-actions will offend us, t-h-I-n-k before you act! Ask yourself, would you want someone to say what your are saying or do what you are doing to your mother? How about our grandmother, wife, sister or daughter? Would you be comfortable in standing up in front of your church congregation saying it or doing it? Finally, ask yourself, "Are my actions becoming of a man?"

Brothers, we love you, we need you and we yearn for your return. Stop turning your backs on the womb that gave you birth. Our children are dying and without our unified spiritual commitment to save ourselves, we will rapidly move from the endangered species category to the category of extinction. Excuses just won't do anymore!

Come back home brothers! A house divided against itself cannot stand.

With Sisterly Love

Patricia Wingard Carson

> PS ...there are countless responsible, strong Black men who have made tremendous sacrifices. And for that, I want to say thank you for standing under the weights of life. Your manhood and leadership are appreciated.
>
> And to my brothers who are incarcerated, you have a greater opportunity to help one another than in any other setting outside of your cell, for you are many under one roof. Start with where you are, with what you have, and be a living example of your kingliness to one another. Then, for those of you who have children, reach beyond the bars of your cell and make your love known to your child. Leave nothing to assumptions. And most importantly, remember that through your Creator, you are magnificently made, wonderfully blessed, and powerfully endowed. Greatness is within you. Don't give up on yourself and don't be too hard on yourself. Learn from your mistakes and move forward to do the good, just, and righteous things that are before you everyday. It will help to keep you strong in spirit, mind, and body.

Each one teach one -- We are all in the same boat and it will take all of our efforts to stay afloat.

To contact the author for seminars, workshops, or training, write to:

Patricia Wingard Carson
Motivational Institute, Inc.
P.O. Box 328712
Colulmbus, Ohio 43232

O R D E R   F O R M   F O R   *P E C U L I A R   P A I N*

Call 1-800-228-0810 to order by telephone or Fax 1-800-772-9165.
Prepayment is required.

- -

YES! I wish to order_____ copies of *Peculiar Pain,* at $24.00
each, plus $3.50 shipping and handling per book.
ISBN #_____.

[ ] Check enclosed [ ] Charge my account

[ ] Master Card   [ ] American Express   [ ] Visa

MC Bank #___/___/___/___   Epiration date: ___/___/___

Account # ___/___/___/___/___/___/___/___/___/___/___/___/___/___/___

Signature _____ (required for all charges)

Name:_____

Phone: (_____) _____

Address:_____

_____

City/State/Zip_____

_____

Make checks payable to: **Kendall/Hunt Publishing Company**
                                        4050 Westmark Drive
                                        Dubuque, Iowa 52004-1840

Special discount rates available when ordered in bulk quantities.
Contact 614-276-5155 for information.